The Many Faces of Depression in Children and Adolescents

Review of Psychiatry Series
John M. Oldham, M.D., M.S.
Michelle B. Riba, M.D., M.S.
Series Editors

The Many Faces of Depression in Children and Adolescents

EDITED BY

David Shaffer, F.R.C.P.(Lond), F.R.C.Psych.(Lond)

Bruce D. Waslick, M.D.

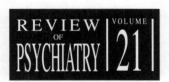

REVIEW OF PSYCHIATRY

VOLUME 21

No. 2

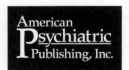

American Psychiatric Publishing, Inc.

Washington, DC
London, England

Note: The authors have worked to ensure that all information in this book concerning drug dosages, schedules, and routes of administration is accurate as of the time of publication and consistent with standards set by the U.S. Food and Drug Administration and the general medical community. As medical research and practice advance, however, therapeutic standards may change. For this reason and because human and mechanical errors sometimes occur, we recommend that readers follow the advice of a physician who is directly involved in their care or the care of a member of their family. A product's current package insert should be consulted for full prescribing and safety information.

ESKIND BIOMEDICAL LIBRARY

JUN 0 7 2002

VANDERBILT UNIVERSITY
NASHVILLE, TN 37232-8340

American Psychiatric Publishing, Inc.
1400 K Street, N.W.
Washington, DC 20005
www.appi.org

The correct citation for this book is

Shaffer D, Waslick BD (editors): *The Many Faces of Depression in Children and Adolescents* (Review of Psychiatry Series, Volume 21, Number 2; Oldham JM and Riba MB, series editors). Washington, DC, American Psychiatric Publishing, 2002

Library of Congress Cataloging-in-Publication Data
The many faces of depression in children and adolescents / edited by David Shaffer, Bruce D. Waslick.
     p. ; cm. — (Review of psychiatry ; v. 21, no. 2)
    Includes bibliographical references and index.
    ISBN 1-58562-071-8 (alk. paper)
    1. Depression in children. 2. Depression in adolescents. 3. Children
Mental health. 4. Teenagers—Mental health. I. Shaffer, David. II. Waslick,
Bruce D. 1960– III. Review of psychiatry series ; v. 21, no. 2.
    [DNLM: 1. Depressive Disorder—therapy—Adolescence. 2. Depressive
Disorder—therapy—Child. 3. Antidepressive Agents—therapeutic use.
4. Depressive Disorder—drug therapy—Adolescence. 5. Depressive Disorder—
drug therapy—Child. 6. Psychotherapy—methods—Adolescence.
7. Psychotherapy—methods—Child. 8. Suicide, Attempted—Adolescence.
9. Suicide, Attempted—Child. WM 171 M2945 2002]
RJ506.D4 M28 2002
618.92'8527—dc21

2001056748

British Library Cataloguing in Publication Data
A CIP record is available from the British Library.

Contents

Chapter 1

**Depression in Children and Adolescents:
An Overview**

Chapter 2

**Psychotherapy for Depression and
Suicidal Behavior in Children and Adolescents**

Contributors

Boris Birmaher, M.D.
Professor of Psychiatry, University of Pittsburgh Medical Center, Western Psychiatric Institute and Clinic, Pittsburgh, Pennsylvania

David Brent, M.D.
Professor of Psychiatry, Pediatrics, and Epidemiology, University of Pittsburgh Medical Center, Western Psychiatric Institute and Clinic, Pittsburgh, Pennsylvania

Gabrielle A. Carlson, M.D.
Professor of Psychiatry and Pediatrics and Director, Child and Adolescent Psychiatry, State University of New York—Stony Brook, Stony Brook, New York

Ted Greenberg, M.P.H.
Research Associate, Columbia University, New York, New York

Aphrodite Kakouros, B.S.
Research Assistant, New York State Psychiatric Institute, New York, New York

Rachel Kandel, B.A.
Research Assistant, New York State Psychiatric Institute, New York, New York

Laura Mufson, Ph.D.
Associate Professor of Clinical Psychology in Psychiatry, College of Physicians and Surgeons, Columbia University, New York, New York

John M. Oldham, M.D., M.S.
Dollard Professor and Acting Chairman, Department of Psychiatry, Columbia University College of Physicians and Surgeons, New York, New York

Michelle B. Riba, M.D., M.S.
Associate Chair for Education and Academic Affairs, Department of Psychiatry, University of Michigan Medical School, Ann Arbor, Michigan

David Shaffer, F.R.C.P.(Lond), F.R.C.Psych.(Lond)
Irving Philips Professor of Child Psychiatry, Columbia University;
Director, Division of Child and Adolescent Psychiatry, New York State
Psychiatric Institute, New York, New York

Drew M. Velting, Ph.D.
Assistant Professor of Clinical Psychology in Psychiatry, College of
Physicians and Surgeons, Columbia University, New York, New York

Bruce D. Waslick, M.D.
Assistant Professor of Clinical Psychiatry, Division of Child Psychiatry,
New York State Psychiatric Institute/Columbia University, New York,
New York

Introduction to the Review of Psychiatry Series

John M. Oldham, M.D., M.S.
Michelle B. Riba, M.D., M.S., Series Editors

2002 REVIEW OF PSYCHIATRY SERIES TITLES

- *Cutting-Edge Medicine: What Psychiatrists Need to Know*
  EDITED BY NADA L. STOTLAND, M.D., M.P.H.
- *The Many Faces of Depression in Children and Adolescents*
  EDITED BY DAVID SHAFFER, F.R.C.P.(LOND), F.R.C.PSYCH.(LOND),
  AND BRUCE D. WASLICK, M.D.
- *Emergency Psychiatry*
  EDITED BY MICHAEL H. ALLEN, M.D.
- *Mental Health Issues in Lesbian, Gay, Bisexual, and Transgender Communities*
  EDITED BY BILLY E. JONES, M.D., M.S., AND MARJORIE J. HILL, PH.D.

There is a growing literature describing the stress–vulnerability model of illness, a model applicable to many, if not most, psychiatric disorders and to physical illness as well. Vulnerability comes in a number of forms. Genetic predisposition to specific conditions may arise as a result of spontaneous mutations, or it may be transmitted intergenerationally in family pedigrees. Secondary types of vulnerability may involve susceptibility to disease caused by the weakened resistance that accompanies malnutrition, immunocompromised states, and other conditions. In most of these models of illness, vulnerability consists of a necessary but not sufficient precondition; if specific stresses are avoided, or if they are encountered but offset by adequate protective factors, the disease does not manifest itself and the vulnerability may never be recognized. Conversely, there is increasing recognition of the role of stress as a precipitant of frank illness in vulnerable individuals and of the complex and subtle interactions among the environment, emotions, and neurodevelopmental, metabolic, and physiological processes.

In this country, the years 2001 and 2002 contained stress of unprecedented proportions, with the terrorist attacks on September 11 and the events that followed that terrible day. Although the contents of Volume 21 of the Review of Psychiatry were well established by that date and much of the text had already been written, we could not introduce this volume without thinking about the relevance of this unanticipated, widespread stress to the topics already planned.

Certainly, major depression is one of the prime candidates among the disorders in vulnerable populations that can be precipitated by stress. The information presented in *The Many Faces of Depression in Children and Adolescents*, edited by David Shaffer and Bruce D. Waslick, is, then, timely indeed. Already identified as a growing problem in youth—all too often accompanied by suicidal behavior—depression in children and adolescents is especially important to identify as early as possible. School-based screening services need to be widespread in order to facilitate both prevention of the disorder in those at risk and referral for effective treatment for those already experiencing symptomatic depression. Both psychotherapy and pharmacotherapy are well established as effective treatments for this condition, making recognition of its presence even more important. In New York alone, thousands of children lost at least one parent in the World Trade Center disaster, a catastrophic event precipitating not just grief but also major depression in the children and adolescents at risk.

We now know that stress, and depression itself, affect not just the brain but the body as well. New information about this brain–body axis is provided in *Cutting-Edge Medicine: What Psychiatrists Need to Know*, edited by Nada L. Stotland. Depression as an independent risk factor for cardiac death is one of the new findings reviewed in the chapter on the mind and the heart, as we understand more about the interactions among emotions, behavior, and cardiovascular functioning. Similarly, stress and mood are primary players in the homeostasis, or lack of it, of other body systems, such as the menstrual cycle and gastrointestinal functioning, also reviewed in this book. Finally, the massive increase in organ transplantation, in which medical advances have made it possible to neutralize the body's own immune responses against foreign tissue, represents a new frontier in which emotional stability is critical in donor and recipient.

Increasingly, medicine's front door is the hospital emergency service. Not just a place where triage occurs, though that remains an important and challenging function, the psychiatric emergency service needs to have expert clinicians who can perform careful assessments and initiate treatment. The latest thinking by psychiatrists experienced in emergency work is presented in *Emergency Psychiatry*, edited by Michael H. Allen. Certainly, psychiatric emergency services serve as one of the most critical components of the response network that needs to be in place to deal with a disaster such as the September 2001 attack and the bioterrorism events that followed.

Perhaps less obviously linked to those September events, *Mental Health Issues in Lesbian, Gay, Bisexual, and Transgender Communities*, edited by Billy E. Jones and Marjorie J. Hill, which reviews current thinking about gay, lesbian, bisexual, and transgender issues, reflects our changing world in other ways. A continuing process is necessary as we rethink our assumptions and challenge and question any prejudice or bias that may have infiltrated our thinking or may have been embedded in our traditional concepts. In this book, traditional notions are contrasted with newer thinking about gender role and sexual orientation, considering these issues from youth to old age, as we continue to try to differentiate the wide range of human diversity from what we classify as illness.

We believe that the topics covered in Volume 21 are timely and represent a selection of important updates for the practicing clinician. Next year, this tradition will continue, with books on trauma and disaster response and management, edited by Robert J. Ursano and Ann E. Norwood; on molecular neurobiology for the clinician, edited by Dennis S. Charney; on geriatric psychiatry, edited by Alan M. Mellow; and on standardized assessment for the clinician, edited by Michael B. First.

Chapter 1

Depression in Children and Adolescents

An Overview

Bruce D. Waslick, M.D.
Rachel Kandel, B.A.
Aphrodite Kakouros, B.S.

As has been the case with many psychiatric disorders, research in pediatric mood disorders required a definition of generally accepted operationalized criteria to make major progress. Before the publication of DSM-III (American Psychiatric Association 1980), prevailing attitudes toward the diagnosis of mood disorders in children and adolescents ranged from the disbelief that these disorders existed prior to later adolescence to overinclusion of many different types of emotional and behavioral disturbances as reflecting *masked depressive reactions*. Masked depressions could be diagnosed in youths manifesting hyperactivity, aggressive behavior, or delinquency if the children or adolescents at times displayed depressed affect and showed depressive or pessimistic themes on projective tests (Cytryn and McKnew 1972).

Because many of the samples of depressed children in the research literature from the 1970s included percentages of children with masked depressions (which today would be considered as primary diagnostic entities distinct from, or comorbid with, depressive illness), it would be fair to say that modern research in pediatric unipolar depressive illness began with the dissemination of the operationalized diagnostic criteria for depressive illness and for other psychiatric diagnoses of childhood in DSM-III (Cytryn et al. 1980). The establishment of operationalized criteria paved the way for the development of diagnostic instruments that could be shared throughout the scientific community. The introduction of these new diagnostic instruments to research with clinical and community samples allowed for some degree of uniformity of diagnostic classification across research groups. Further refinement of the instruments, as well as their use in larger samples of children and adolescents, allowed descriptive efforts, which took the first steps toward defining pediatric depressive disorders as illnesses of consequence by describing consistent symptomatic presentations, documenting associated impairment, investigating risk factors for illness, and characterizing the natural history and clinical course of the disorder.

The following overview is meant to summarize important research regarding the clinical description, diagnosis, epidemiology, etiology, and natural history of depressive disorders in children and adolescents. In this chapter, we focus on unipolar depressive disorders because bipolar disorders are covered elsewhere in this volume. No topic can be covered exhaustively, but important concepts emerging from recent empirical efforts to describe and understand the cause of depressive illness in children are highlighted. Other chapters in this volume report more extensively on intervention approaches and research, but treatment implications of the topics covered in this chapter are noted.

Clinical Description

Depression in children and adolescents can present as a component of many different clinical problems that are common reasons for referral to mental health professionals. Some of the more common clinical presentations are listed in this section, although the list is not intended to be exhaustive. The clinical problems described in this section may seem very different and unlikely to be related, but research evidence is available for the association of depressive illness in youth with each clinical problem in this section. It should be understood that not all children manifesting the problems described below will in fact have a diagnosable mood disorder, so that each clinical presentation is not specifically associated with depressive illness alone. The presence of other mental health disorders of childhood may need to be considered by clinicians assessing patients presenting with the problems described.

Distinct and Enduring Mood Change

Children and adolescents referred for evaluation may present primarily with a recognizable onset of distressing or impairing mood symptoms (Puig-Antich and Weston 1983). Parents and other adults who come into frequent contact with a particular child may notice a general change in the child's mood state or demeanor. Dysphoria and/or irritability may take the place of contentment and euthymia as the child's predominating mood state. Parents may notice increasing levels of unhappiness, tearfulness, anger reactions, or frank rages set off by minimal or minor provocations in their child. The changes in a child's affective tone and emotional regulatory capacity, which eventually may be diagnosed as manifestations of clinical depression, generally go beyond childhood or adolescent moodiness. States of distinct mood changes lasting more than a few days are of more significant concern than a brief day or two of feeling down or irritable. Parents, especially those with personal or family histories of depression, may recognize early signs of a developing mood disorder and may seek consultation. Rarely do children or adolescents seek, on their own, contact with mental health professionals for evaluation of developing mood symptoms, although they may more frequently make contact with available professionals or services located on-site in school settings. Therefore, it may be of increasingly greater importance to provide school-based professionals with education about the signs and symptoms of depressive illness so as to increase the likelihood of early recognition and appropriate intervention for youths with mood disorders.

School Problems

Common co-occurring problems for depressed children and adolescents are academic underachievement, school attendance problems, and school failure (Hammen et al. 1999). Although it is often presumed that the co-occurring problems are consequences of depression in youths, academic problems can precede the onset of depressive symptoms for some children. It is generally recognized that cognitive components of depressive syndromes make it exceedingly difficult for children, adolescents, and adults to fully maintain their normal level of academic and vocational functioning. Young persons with depression often experience problems with decreasing levels of subjective interest in academic progress, difficulty concentrating and paying attention in class and during homework periods, and loss of the necessary energy and motivation levels that are required for academic achievement, making premorbid levels of school functioning increasingly difficult to maintain. At times, some individuals become so impaired that they may abandon their hopes of attaining any academic achievement or success and even withdraw entirely from attending school, making clinical depression one of the more common psychiatric diagnoses identifiable in populations of school refusers (King and Bernstein 2001).

Family Conflict

Increasing levels of family conflict are a common referral reason for families of depressed youths (Hammen et al. 1999). Irritability in the child may lead to frequent unpleasant interactions with parents or siblings. Conflicts may arise over the child's increasing academic problems, and parents can become alarmed, concerned, or, frequently, angry about deteriorating school performance. Familial role disputes may arise when a child disabled by severe depression may be unable to maintain functioning in certain types of roles previously assigned to, or taken on by, the child. Adolescents dealing with depressive symptoms often will instinctively try to find ways to cope with their increasing dysphoria, which can include activities (e.g., overinvesting time and energy with certain peer groups, avoiding taxing school assignments, experimenting with sexual activity and illicit substance use) that adults may consider problematic or unhealthy, at times prompting a referral for evaluation.

Suicidal Crises

It is not uncommon, especially in adolescents, for the initial presenting problem bringing a depressed minor into contact with a health professional to be a suicidal crisis. The crisis can be the result of the youth's direct or indirect expression of suicidal thoughts or ideas, or of actually engaging in some form of self-harming behavior, ranging from nonsuicidal self-injury (e.g., superficially scratching the skin of the wrists) to severe, life-threatening suicide attempts accompanied by the express wish to bring about death. Although not all children or adolescents presenting with a suicidal crisis have a mood disorder, depression is a leading risk factor for suicidal ideation and attempts (Gould et al. 1998), as well as for completed suicide (Shaffer et al. 1996b), in both prepubertal and adolescent populations. Evaluation for the presence of mood disorder is therefore an essential component of a crisis evaluation for all suicidal youth.

Increasing Illicit Substance Abuse

Mood symptoms can precede, co-occur with, or follow periods of illicit substance use or abuse in children and adolescents (Costello et al. 1999; Kandel et al. 1999). Depressed youths often seek means of alleviating their increasing levels of dysphoria by experimenting, or regularly intoxicating themselves, with illicit substances. Marijuana use and abuse among depressed adolescents are common, and discovery of marijuana use by adult authorities or parental figures may direct the involved child to some type of mental health evaluation or intervention. Although it appears that, in many case series, most youths presenting to substance abuse treatment centers do not have primary mood disorders (e.g., Garland et al. 2001), a sizable minority of patients do in fact report clinical levels of depression. These patients may need an intervention plan that differs from that for patients without concurrent mood disorder.

Somatic Symptoms

Depressed children and adolescents commonly present to health care professionals with physical symptoms (Ryan et al. 1987), such as headache, chronic fatigue, gastrointestinal symptoms, and musculoskeletal aches and pains. School nurses and primary care physicians may be called on to evaluate somatic symptoms that may be related to depressive illness in youths. In addition, depression can be a comorbid condition, or a complication, of medical illness or medical treatment in youths. Depression is often present in children and adolescents with diabetes mellitus (e.g., Goldston et al. 1994) and other medical illnesses. Depression sometimes can be associated with certain types of medical therapies, such as phenobarbital treatment of epilepsy (Brent et al. 1990) or the use of isotretinoin for acne (Hull and Demkiw-Bartel 2000).

Diagnosis

Making an accurate diagnosis of a mood disorder, or any mental health syndrome, in children and adolescents is a complicated task that may require considerable training and experience.

Diagnostic Criteria

For years it was believed and taught that children and adolescents could not have mood disorders and that clinical depression was a syndrome that required a minimal level of developmental achievement before one could truly be given the diagnosis of the disorder. Operationalized criteria defined in the 1970s and 1980s for depressive syndromes in adults were applied to younger patients, and investigators consistently found that children and adolescents reported similar concurrent constellations of emotional, cognitive, and behavioral symptoms that were, for all practical purposes, difficult to distinguish from adult depressive syndromes.

In general, as the various editions of DSM began to take root as the primary diagnostic reference in American psychiatry, the diagnostic criteria for mood disorders were established as essentially uniform across the developmental spectrum. Currently, in DSM-IV-TR (American Psychiatric Association 2000), one uses essentially the same diagnostic criteria for making a diagnosis of a major depressive episode in young children as one does in adults and the elderly, with two exceptions. First, the primary mood state has been modified for children and adolescents to allow inclusion of irritable mood as a depressive equivalent in youths, whereas in adults and the elderly, irritability is not considered a specific diagnostic criterion that would contribute to the diagnosis of depression (although certainly anger and irritability may be components of the clinical presentation of the disorder in a proportion of depressed adults). Second, rather than maintaining strict adherence to a weight loss criterion for children and adolescents, because it is expected that a normally developing child or adolescent will continue to grow in body size throughout most of adolescence, DSM-IV-TR specifies that a pediatric patient can meet the appetite and weight disruption criterion by failing to maintain normally expected growth and weight gains. In all other operationalized criteria for a major depressive episode, adult and youth diagnostic criteria are identical.

Researchers examining the symptomatic presentation of depressed youths compared with adults have concluded that, for the most part, symptom patterns for depression are largely similar across the developmental spectrum in both clinical and community samples (Kovacs 1996; Lewinsohn et al. 1998). Children appear to rarely have hypersomnia during depressive episodes, and children and adolescents may be less susceptible to psychotic symptoms such as delusions during the course of a depressive episode when compared with adults and the elderly; in general, however, symptomatic presentation is not readily distinguishable between youths and adults (Kovacs 1996).

Developmental Issues

In clinical practice, although the operationalized criteria for making a diagnosis of a depressive disorder in youths and adults are very similar, the process of a diagnostic evaluation is somewhat different. For diagnostic evaluation of an adult patient, primary emphasis is generally placed on the interview with the identified patient. With children and adolescents, much greater emphasis must be placed on collateral sources of information. These collateral sources may include interviews with parents, discussions with school officials and teachers, reports or records from the child's primary health care provider, and interviews with other concerned family members or adults who are well informed about the child's life and habits. Additionally, diagnostic evaluation is complicated by limitations in the cognitive or verbal abilities of younger patients. Young children may have difficulty recognizing and understanding the meaning of some symptoms as well as in communicating their emotional and psychological experience to others. Some diagnostic criteria may be exceedingly difficult to assess at certain developmental stages. For instance, awareness of more complex cognitive symptoms such as guilt or a deficient capacity for making decisions may be easily reportable by adults and older adolescents but may be difficult to identify in preschool and latency-aged children and some young adolescents.

One ongoing problem in research on psychiatric diagnosis in children and adolescents is the common occurrence of parent-child disagreement during assessment for diagnostic criteria, and this problem certainly is evident in the research literature for pediatric mood disorders (Andrews et al. 1993). Studies assessing mood disorder prevalence can give very different prevalence rates depending on whether the diagnosis is made on the basis of the youth informant, the parent informant, or some algorithm combining the two informants. Some research groups (e.g., Lewinsohn et al. 1993) essentially ignored parent information when assessing samples of older adolescents, especially when the primary research questions centered on internalizing disorders such as depression. Other studies tried to incorporate both parent and child information but found minimal agreement between informants and therefore reported overall depression prevalence rates at nearly twice the rate of single informant rates (Garrison et al. 1992; Shaffer et al. 1996a).

Current preference among researchers is to err on the side of using an "OR" rule, in which a symptom or diagnosis is counted as present if either the parent or the child informant reports that it is present because it is assumed that both parties contribute meaningful data to the assessment (Bird et al. 1992). An alternative strategy would be to use an "AND" rule, in which a diagnosis is counted only if both the child and the parent agree on the presence of the disorder, but this strategy would yield very low prevalence rates of mood disorders in most studies.

Diagnostic assessment problems are further complicated by the fact that the presence or absence of a psychiatric diagnosis in a parent can influence his or her reporting of psychiatric symptoms in the child. For example, Renouf and Kovacs (1994) found clear evidence that the presence of depression in mothers was associated with a greater degree of mother-child disagreement in reports of depressive symptomatology present in the child because depressed mothers consistently overrated their child's symptom levels compared with the child's self-reports.

Comorbidity

Only a minority of cases of depressive disorders in youths seen in clinical practice may be uncomplicated by other Axis I or Axis II disorders (Kovacs 1996). Community samples also detect high rates of comorbidity of depressive disorders with other disorders (Bird et al. 1993; Lewinsohn et al. 1995). Studies with both community and clinical samples of depressed youths show that referred children with mood disorders commonly have a variety of other concurrent diagnoses, including anxiety disorders, disruptive behavior disorders, substance abuse or dependence, eating disorders, and learning disabilities. In addition, comorbidity of mood disorders with medical problems is not uncommon.

Some studies have suggested that youths with depressive disorders presenting concurrently with other types of psychiatric symptoms may have more impairment than do youths with more "pure" unipolar depressions (e.g., Lewinsohn et al. 1995). Comorbidity may complicate treatment planning because certain comorbid conditions have, in some treatment studies, predicted worse short-term clinical response. In addition, adult outcomes of depressed youths may vary depending on the presence or absence of concurrent nonaffective psychiatric disorders. For example, the presence of certain comorbid disorders, such as conduct disorder, in subgroups of depressed youths has predicted poorer long-term outcome when these groups were compared with subjects with relatively uncomplicated depressive illness (Harrington et al. 1991).

Research Issues

Diagnostic Instruments

Instruments used to diagnose the presence or absence of a depressive disorder are available for use with children and adolescents. Diagnostic instruments commonly cited in the research literature are listed in Table 1–1. For all practical purposes, the instruments can be divided along several different parameters, including the types of samples in which the instrument was designed to be used (community vs. clinical), the degree of structuring of the assessment questions (highly structured "yes-or-no" questions vs. open-ended clinical inquiry), and whether the interview was designed to be administered by individuals with minimal or extensive instrument-specific or professional training. For example, some instruments, such as the Diagnostic Interview Schedule for Children (DISC), were developed primarily for use in epidemiological research on various disorders of childhood and adolescence, in which large numbers of children and adolescents were to be assessed with the instrument in a cost-effective manner to ascertain information such as prevalence and disease burden in a given community. These instruments tend to be highly structured and offer little room for interpretive work by the interviewer administering the instrument. Lay interviewers can be trained to use the instrument and are not required to have extensive clinical training. Other instruments, such as the Schedule for Affective Disorders and Schizophrenia for School-Aged Children (K-SADS), were developed to be administered by clinically trained diagnosticians and may be used more often in research with clinical samples. Characteristics of diagnostic instruments used in mood disorder studies commonly referenced in the pediatric psychiatry literature are also presented in Table 1–1.

In addition, instruments assessing symptomatic severity of depressive symptoms in children and adolescents are available

Table 1–1. Diagnostic instruments commonly used in pediatric depression research

Diagnostic instrument	Degree of structure to instrument	Minimal qualifications to administer	Test-retest reliability for MDD	Interrater reliability for MDD	Application to research on MDD
Diagnostic Interview Schedule for Children, Version IV (DISC-IV; Shaffer et al. 2000)	Highly structured	Lay interviewers with some training (2–3 days)	Fair	High	Epidemiological work mostly
Child and Adolescent Psychiatric Assessment (CAPA; Angold and Costello 2000)	Highly structured	Lay interviewers with more training (2–4 weeks)	Good	High	Epidemiological work mostly
Diagnostic Interview for Children and Adolescents (DICA; Reich 2000)	Highly structured	Lay interviewers with more training (2–4 weeks)	Fair in children, better in adolescents	High	Epidemiological work mostly
Schedule for Affective Disorders and Schizophrenia for School-Aged Children (K-SADS; Ambrosini 2000)	Semistructured	Trained clinician	Good	Good	Epidemiological work, family studies, treatment research

Table 1–1. Diagnostic instruments commonly used in pediatric depression research *(continued)*

Diagnostic instrument	Degree of structure to instrument	Minimal qualifications to administer	Test-retest reliability for MDD	Interrater reliability for MDD	Application to research on MDD
Interview Schedule for Children and Adolescents (ISCA; Sherrill and Kovacs 2000)	Semistructured	Trained clinician	Good	Good	Longitudinal research in naturalistic studies
Children's Interview for Psychiatric Syndromes (ChIPS; Weller et al. 2000)	Structured	Trained lay interviewers	Not available	Good	Screening for mental disorders in clinical or community samples

Note. MDD=major depressive disorder.

for a wide variety of research purposes, ranging from use as screening instruments in population surveys to scales serving to document change in symptomatic severity in treatment studies. Some instruments, such as the Hamilton Rating Scale for Depression and the Beck Depression Inventory, were developed to be used in adult samples and have been introduced as measures in children and adolescents essentially unmodified. Others, such as the Children's Depression Rating Scale and the self-rated Children's Depression Inventory, were developed in novel formats to be used in research with pediatric populations. A list of commonly used instruments assessing depression severity is included in Table 1–2.

Measurement Issues

Measurement issues in research on pediatric mood disorders are of primary importance for the field as a whole. To be of significant value in advancing research into the epidemiology, etiology, natural history, and treatment of mood disorders, instruments must validly and reliably assess both the presence and the absence of disorder as well as precisely measure the severity of disorder. Precision of measurement is notoriously difficult to achieve in mental health research because of the absence of a physically measurable process relating to "mood problems" that can be quantified. However, instruments can be developed to show reasonable standards of test-retest and interrater reliability as well as internal consistency.

Psychometric studies of currently available diagnostic instruments and severity scales are available for most of the instruments listed in Tables 1–1 and 1–2. In general, most of the diagnostic instruments available have fair to good test-retest and interrater reliability for depressive disorders in youths, and the severity scales that are currently available have reasonable evidence supporting reliability and validity for use in research on depressed youths. It would be difficult to recommend any one instrument above and beyond any other based on currently available data on the instruments and measures themselves. Selection of instruments for use in any given research endeavor should primarily take into account instrument characteristics and record of

Table 1–2. Depressive symptom rating scales used in pediatric depression research

Instrument	Format	Appropriate ages (years)	Application
Children's Depression Inventory (CDI; Kovacs 1981)	Self-administered	8–12	Depression screening, self-rated symptom scale
Center for Epidemiologic Studies Depression Scale (CES-D; Garrison et al. 1991)	Self-administered	8–17	Screen for depression in large samples
Reynolds Adolescent Depression Scale (RADS; Reynolds 1998)	Self-administered	12–17	Self-rated symptom scale, treatment research as a measure of change
Beck Depression Inventory (BDI; Beck et al. 1961)	Self-administered	12–17	Self-rated symptom scale, treatment research as a measure of change
Children's Depression Rating Scale (CDRS; Poznanski et al. 1979)	Semistructured interview	6–18	Depression screening, treatment research
Schedule for Affective Disorders and Schizophrenia for School-Aged Children (K-SADS) 17-item subscale (e.g., Ambrosini et al. 1991)	Semistructured interview	6–18	Depression severity rating
Hamilton Rating Scale for Depression (Hamilton 1967)	Structured interview	12–18	Depression severity rating, treatment research as a measure of change

use of the instrument in similar study designs and populations, in concert with an independent assessment of psychometric properties of chosen instruments in preparatory work for a research project.

Validity Issues

Establishing a diagnostic instrument as valid—meaning that the instrument is measuring what the user is intending to measure—is different from establishing that what the instrument is measuring is in fact a valid and specific "illness" or "disorder." Because most diagnostic instruments try to assess for the presence or absence of operationalized criteria (currently, mainly signs or symptoms) established for a disorder, and do so by having the interviewer either observe whether a sign is present or essentially ask the patient (or others who know the patient) whether a symptom exists, most diagnostic instruments available for use in pediatric samples today have relatively good face validity (McClellan and Werry 2000).

It is not quite so simple to establish that the syndrome that an instrument is trying to assess is in fact a valid illness. According to the approach set out by Robins and Guze (1970), determining that a diagnostic entity is in fact a valid illness requires 1) adequate clinical description of the illness, including delineating symptoms, suffering, and morbidity; 2) correlation of the illness to laboratory studies, if possible; 3) demarcation of the illness from other illnesses and subsyndromal illness; and 4) determination that the illness follows a predictable clinical course via longitudinal observation. (Robins and Guze also recommended establishing familiality of a disorder, which certainly is appropriate for illnesses with genetic correlates, but one would hardly argue that lobar pneumonia is not an illness in a given individual because it does not appear to be familial in a given population.)

Validity of a diagnostic entity as an illness initially can be inferred if the clinical description depicts consistent symptomatic presentations and meaningful suffering and impairment. But clinical description also should distinguish specific features of the illness that warrant classifying it differently from other types of illness (e.g., because the diagnosis differentially predicts clinical course or response to certain interventions compared with other syndromes or illnesses). Beyond clinical description, validity of a disorder can be further demonstrated if specific etiological factors can be identified; quantified by physical, chemical, or other types of laboratory instrumentation; and controlled to alter the onset or clinical course of the illness and if the longitudinally determined natural history of the illness confirms future morbidity or mortality.

There is little doubt that children and adolescents meeting criteria for major depression, whether ascertained from clinical or community samples, experience significant concurrent functional impairment in several domains (i.e., academic, health, social). High levels of comorbidity, however, do call into question the specificity of the diagnosis because dysphoric reactions, even when prolonged, sometimes can be attributable to a variety of negative events and stresses. In addition, groups of individuals with subsyndromal depressive symptoms that do not meet criteria for the diagnosis of major depression have shown in some studies similar levels of impairment and similar longitudinal course of illness as those meeting full criteria (Lewinsohn et al. 2000). No specific laboratory tests are available to diagnose depressive illness at any developmental stage. In addition, as described later in this chapter (see "Natural History and Clinical Course"), there is a fair amount of discontinuity between depressive disorders arising in childhood and mood disorders in adults, especially in cases of prepubertal-onset depression. Outcomes for individuals with childhood-onset depressive illness vary, with a percentage of subjects in any given study having very good outcomes, others having prolonged problems with affective illness, and still others developing other types of nonaffective psychiatric illness. Therefore, ongoing research is needed to further refine diagnostic criteria to improve construct and predictive validity of depressive illness in youths, and to develop laboratory tests that can be used as independent validators of mood disorder in afflicted patients.

Epidemiology

Prevalence

The point prevalence of depressive disorders in community samples of children and adolescents varies as a function of the instrument used, the sampling process, the age range of the population sampled, and whether the target population is a true community sample or a school-based sample. Table 1–3 lists several studies that attempted to assess the point prevalence of depressive disorders in community samples of children and adolescents as well as the ascertained prevalence rates. In general, the point prevalence of depression ranges from about 1% to 3% in prepubertal children and from 3% to 9% in adolescents, attesting to the fact that advancing age is a risk factor for the onset of depression in youth. Although no clear difference in prevalence rates was found between sexes in prepubertal samples, females have been consistently identified as being at higher risk for depression after the onset of puberty. Studies generally have reported that females are twice as likely to have depressive illness by later adolescence compared with males, and this sex ratio is generally maintained throughout most of adulthood. Few studies have assessed large enough samples of minority youths to give precise estimates of prevalence differences varying by race/ethnicity. Low socioeconomic status also has been shown to be a risk factor for many types of psychiatric disorders in children and adolescents, including mood disorders (e.g., Costello et al. 1996).

Most studies in Table 1–3 reported on only point prevalence of disorder. Lewinsohn et al. (1993) also assessed lifetime prevalence rates of depressive disorders in their sample of older adolescents and found that approximately 20%–25% of the adolescents reported a lifetime history of at least one episode of major depression, whereas 3% of the adolescents reported a lifetime history of dysthymic disorder.

Incidence

Few studies have attempted to ascertain, through longitudinal sampling, the incidence rate of depressive disorders in youths,

Table 1–3. Major epidemiological assessments of the prevalence of depressive disorder in youths

Study	Sample characteristics	Diagnostic method or instrument	Point prevalence of MDD
Fleming et al. 1989	Community-based; ages 6–16	Survey Diagnostic Instrument/DSM-III checklists (6-month prevalence)	Children: 0.6% Adolescents: 1.8%
Whitaker et al. 1990	School-based; grades 9–12	Initial screen, then DSM-III checklist	4%
McGee et al. 1990	Birth cohort; age 15	Diagnostic Interview Schedule for Children (DISC-C)	1.2%
Garrison et al. 1992	School-based; ages 12–14	Initial screen, then Schedule for Affective Disorders and Schizophrenia for School-Aged Children (K-SADS)	9.0%
Cohen et al. 1993	Community-based; ages 10–20	Diagnostic Interview Schedule for Children, Version 1 (DISC-1)	Ages 10–13: 2.0% Ages 14–16: 4.7% Ages 17–20: 2.7%
Lewinsohn et al. 1993	School-based; grades 9–12	K-SADS (no parent information)	2.6%
Fergusson et al. 1993	Birth cohort	DISC-1 (12-month prevalence)	~6.0%
Shaffer et al. 1996a	Community-based; ages 9–17	DISC, Version 2.3 (6-month prevalence rates)	5.6%[a]
Costello et al. 1996	Community-based; ages 9–13	Child and Adolescent Psychiatric Assessment (3-month prevalence rates)	0.03%

Note. MDD=major depressive disorder. [a]Not taking into account any impairment criteria.

and the available published studies assessing incidence primarily targeted adolescent samples. For example, Garrison et al. (1997) found 1-year incidence rates of about 3% for both major depression and dysthymic disorder in their school-based sample of young adolescents aged 11–16 years. Lewinsohn et al. (1993), studying a school-based sample of older high school students, found that adolescents reported a 1-year incidence rate of 8% for major depression and a very low rate of 0.08% for dysthymic disorder. Lewinsohn et al. (1993) found a greater than twofold higher incidence of major depression in females compared with males, but Garrison et al. (1997) found no sex effect on incidence in their younger sample.

Etiology

As with depressive disorders of adulthood, there is no clearly defined single cause of most or even many cases of pediatric depression. Depressive syndromes in youths may in fact be the phenotypic expressions of a final common pathway for several pathological processes, and current attempts at establishing specific etiological cause for most cases generally have not been successful. However, research with pediatric populations has identified several variables that can be considered risk factors or promising etiological correlates. These correlates are approached in this section with a biopsychosocial model, in which biological, psychological, and social/environmental variables identified through research are categorized and briefly described. Some of the identified risk factors operate at the level of relatively nonspecific risk factors for psychopathology, but others have been more specifically linked to depressive disorders in youths.

Biological Correlates

Genetics

Family studies with pediatric samples confirm the familial nature of depressive disorders with child and adolescent probands (Klein et al. 2001; Kovacs et al. 1997; Puig-Antich et al. 1989). Family history studies and family interview studies suggest that depressive disorders occur at higher rates in adult relatives of depressed children and adolescents, and the increased rates of depressive disorders appear to be relatively specific, as opposed to elevated rates of all types of psychiatric disorders. Additionally, "high-risk" studies consistently found that offspring of parents with mood disorders had higher rates of childhood- and adolescent-onset mood disorders than did control subjects (Angold et al. 1987; Weissman et al. 1997). Twin studies with adolescent samples confirmed that monozygous twins have higher rates of concordance for depressive disorders than do dizygous or nontwin siblings (e.g., Eaves et al. 1997). Familiality of a disorder suggests, but is not conclusive evidence of, the presence of a genetic diathesis in cases of pediatric depression because there are other explanations for syndromes aggregating in families that may not be the result of genetics (see subsection "Parenting Considerations" later in this chapter). No specific genetic abnormality or polymorphism has yet been conclusively established to confer an elevated risk of developing unipolar major depression in children, adolescents, or adults.

Temperament

In contemporary child development research, temperament refers to a constitutional style presumably inherited by the child and that to some extent sets the stage for and moderates organism-environment interaction. Observable infant and toddler behaviors such as activity level, adaptability to change and novel stimuli, response intensity to environmental events, and perseverance in the face of obstacles are some of the variables measured observationally or psychometrically in modern child temperament research. The concept that certain childhood temperamental factors may specifically predict psychiatric diagnoses over time is intriguing and has some support, including studies suggesting that a particular temperament termed *behaviorally inhibited* may be associated with the development of anxiety disorders in youths (e.g., Biederman et al. 1993). However, no conclusive evidence now exists to show specific links between temperamental differences and the development of mood disorders in children.

Neuroendocrine Factors

The fact that females become increasingly at risk for developing depression after the onset of puberty has suggested that sex hormones may be associated with mood disorders in a causal manner (Angold et al. 1999). Both males and females undergo many hormonal changes during puberty and adolescence, and some of these changes have been correlated to the increased risk of depression in adolescent females. However, psychological development and socialization of adolescents also diverge during this phase for boys and girls, with girls tending to develop "affiliative" relationship patterns that presage maternal behavior, and boys tending to prefer independence and autonomy (Cyranowski et al. 2000). In association with diverging developmental patterns and neurohormonal changes, other risk factors such as impaired attachment styles, temperamental differences, and increased reactivity to negative life events may combine to explain in a more comprehensive way the sex difference in depression risk that develops during adolescence and is maintained throughout most of adulthood.

Studies examining other endocrine factors and their role in the etiology of childhood depression have had mixed results. In general, assessments of the association of adrenal steroid hypersecretion in prepubertal or adolescent patients with depressive disorders have been equivocal; some studies (Emslie et al. 1987; Weller et al. 1985) supported the idea that dysregulation of adrenal cortisol secretion is associated with childhood depression, but others did not (Birmaher et al. 1992a, 1992b). A few studies have examined the role of thyroid hormone regulation in the etiology of depression in children and adolescents with mixed results (Dorn et al. 1997; Garcia et al. 1991). More extensive work has suggested that dysregulation of the secretion of growth hormone may be associated with pediatric depression (Ryan et al. 1994); it also may possibly be a trait marker for depressive illness in prepubertal children (Birmaher et al. 1997) and adolescents (Birmaher et al. 2000).

Neurotransmitter Studies

Few studies have examined the role of specific neurochemical processes in pediatric populations. Preliminary evidence from studies that used peripheral markers of central catecholamine function, such as blood serotonin levels (Hughes et al. 1996) or platelet serotonin receptors (Sallee et al. 1998), and from neuroendocrine challenge studies with L-5-hydroxytryptophan (Ryan et al. 1992) or m-chlorophenylpiperazine (Ghaziuddin et al. 2000) indicates that central serotonergic function may be altered in subsamples of depressed children and adolescents.

Brain Anatomy

The use of both structural and functional neuroimaging techniques in pediatric samples is a relatively new methodology for attempting to understand the biological correlates of mood disorders. Preliminary evidence for the role of altered brain structure in depressed youths is available for some brain regions, such as the observation that depressed adolescents appear to have reduced frontal lobe volumes compared with healthy control subjects (Steingard et al. 1996). In addition, there have been recent attempts to study functional neuroanatomy with newer neuroimaging techniques. Initial results suggest that alteration in monoamine function or cerebral perfusion in specific brain regions, such as the frontal (Steingard et al. 2000), temporoparietal (Kowatch et al. 1999), or occipital lobes (Bonte et al. 2001), may be associated with mood disorder in youths.

Sleep

Abnormality or irregularity of sleep patterns and sleep physiology has been varyingly studied as a precursor, biological marker, symptom, or consequence of depressive mood problems in youths. Evidence suggests that not getting enough sleep as is physiologically required can lead to alterations in mood state and functional performance in youths (Dahl 1998). Alternatively, it appears likely that the onset of major depression is accompanied by a physiological state in which altered sleep patterns, often characterized by relative insomnia, occur. Sleep study assessments of depressed youths and nondepressed control subjects have yielded inconsistent results. Some studies (Emslie et al. 1990, 1994), but not all (Goetz et al. 1987; Puig-Antich et al. 1982), have reported statistically different sleep characteristics—such as increased sleep latency, shortened rapid eye movement (REM) sleep latency, increased duration of REM sleep overall, and lower percentages of stage 2 and 3 non-REM sleep—that are similar to the findings of studies with depressed adults. Additionally, one study found that dysregulated sleep physiology may be a marker for an increased likelihood of depression recurrence after recovery (Emslie et al. 2001).

Psychological Correlates

Cognitive Factors

Cognitive theories of depression postulate that the presence in an individual of *dysfunctional attitudes,* including a pessimistic view of one's self, world, or future, or *negative attributional style,* in which negative events in one's life are conceptualized as the result of internal (self-related), stable (vs. transient), and global (vs. specific) causes, precedes the development of depressive disorders. These cognitive factors are thought to create a diathesis for depression in youths and adults. Research supporting the presence of these "depressogenic" cognitive abnormalities in patients with depression forms the theoretical basis for the use of cognitive therapies in youths and adults (see Gotlib and Abramson 1999).

Animal models suggest that the behavioral manifestations that have certain features in common with depressive illness in humans can develop in animals that are subjected to negative events from which there is no opportunity to escape. A "learned helplessness" paradigm typically entails the organism being subjected to unwanted events over which it can exert only minimal regulatory control (Seligman 1984). Animals, and potentially humans, placed in circumstances from which no escape is possible can develop passivity to negative life events, which on superficial examination can resemble neurovegetative symptoms of depression, such as psychomotor retardation, listlessness, and loss of goal-directed behavior. It is tempting to correlate this type of animal model to depressive illness, in which an individual can become demoralized when confronted with unescapable negative life events, such as family discord, poverty, learning problems, or peer rejection. Although little direct evidence is available in research with human youths that would support this kind of causal model, depression in youths has been frequently correlated with negative life events (e.g., Lewinsohn et al. 2001).

Negative Life Events

The experience of negative life events usually is thought of as a precipitating factor or stressor in most stress-diathesis models of depression. Negative life events that have been particularly correlated to the onset of depressive symptoms include loss events and failure in goal-directed behaviors. *Loss events,* such as death of a close family member or the breakup of a romantic relationship, have been associated with the onset of major depression in children and adolescents (Monroe et al. 1999). Death of a friend, sibling, or parent from suicide conveys an increased risk for developing major depression and suicidal thinking in the 6 months following the suicide (Brent et al. 1993a, 1993c; Cerel et al. 1999). *Failure events,* such as inability to achieve academic or social goals, may interact with predisposing dysfunctional cognitive schemas to induce and maintain dysphoric states (Lewinsohn et al. 2001).

Child Abuse

The experience of physical and sexual abuse during childhood years has been associated with an increased risk for depression. This is suggested by the results of studies asking adolescents and adults to report retrospectively on memories of their childhood years (Roosa et al. 1999) as well as studies assessing psychiatric symptoms and diagnoses in youths known to have been victims of abuse (Kaufman 1991). Ongoing emotional and physical abuse of children has been postulated as one source of negative attributional styles that develop in individuals at risk for depression and may be a human correlate of inducing the state of learned helplessness in exposed children.

Affective Regulation Deficiencies

Little research has been done on the development of the ability to regulate affective states in children and adolescents. The study of the development of the capacity to regulate one's affective states is an extraordinarily complex research subject. Presumably, research in the development of the capacity to regulate one's affect effectively must take into account brain development, as well as cognitive and affective neuroscience. Models would take into account not only the accurate description of one's negative affect states but also an individual's ability to induce and maintain positive affective states. A preliminary study suggested that depressed youths appear to be less able to terminate negative affect states in a timely manner than are nondepressed comparison groups (Sheeber et al. 2000). However, this result could be state dependent, or alternatively a sequela or "scar," as opposed to an etiological cause, of depression in youths.

Sexual Identity

Various research groups have shown that developing a nonheterosexual sexual identity is associated with a variety of adverse mental health problems, including depression and suicidal behavior (e.g., Fergusson et al. 1999). Gay, lesbian, and bisexual youths, whose sexual orientation is determined either by self-definition or on the basis of reports of sexual interests or behavior, are increasingly being recognized as being at risk for psychiatric distress, although the precise mechanism of this association has yet to be determined. It is not clear if the psychiatric symptoms develop as a result of the stress associated with coming to terms with a minority sexual orientation within one's family or peer culture or by some other mechanism.

Social/Environmental Correlates

Poverty

Poverty and lower socioeconomic status in families have been associated with an increased risk for a variety of mental health problems, including serious emotional disturbance. However, it is generally recognized that poverty is a rather nonspecific risk factor for mental illness, and no studies currently correlate lack of available resources to any one specific type of mental health problem (e.g., Costello et al. 1996).

Parenting Considerations

Parenting behavior can influence the development of depression in youths in many different ways. As noted earlier in this chapter, depression appears to be familial, and parents of depressed youths appear to be at relatively high risk for experiencing depression themselves (Ferro et al. 2000). During depressive episodes, depressed parents may be moody, emotionally volatile, disengaged, difficult to please, and not necessarily capable of monitoring and tending to basic emotional and physical needs of their children. Depressed parents also may model thinking patterns that are filled with cognitive errors, distortions, negativity, and other components that may serve to inoculate their offspring with depressogenic cognitive styles. In addition, highly critical parenting, offering high levels of expressed emotion, may predispose children to developing depressive illness, possibly by leading to correlates of learned helplessness in the face of relentless negative appraisals. A longitudinal study of a community sample by Johnson et al. (2001) suggested that maladaptive parental behavior may, over time, be a nonspecific risk factor for a variety of psychopathological outcomes, including depression, in children and adolescents. In this study, the association between maladaptive parenting behavior and the development of psychopathology was evident even after the presence of parental psychopathology and child temperamental difficulties were controlled for.

Peer Environments

Depressed children and adolescents commonly have difficulties interacting with their same-age peers. Depressed children and adolescents may have more difficulty developing effective social problem-solving skills, leading to a greater chance of being rejected or perceived as less competent in a variety of areas by their peers (e.g., Cole 1990).

Natural History and Clinical Course

Age at Onset

An episode of major depression can present at any developmental age, from the preschool years through adolescence. As described earlier in this chapter, advancing age is a risk factor for the onset of depressive illness in boys and girls, and the peak incidence of depression occurs in the later adolescent years. It appears that the long-term outcome for youths with depression is somewhat different depending on whether onset of illness occurred in the prepubertal years or in adolescence. Longitudinal studies of children with prepubertal onset of depression suggested that those individuals with family histories of depression may be at higher risk for experiencing recurrent depressive episodes and specific impairment from mood disorders (Weissman et al. 1999b). Moreover, in general, prepubertal onset of depression predicts significant psychiatric disorders in adulthood, but the disorders are not specifically related to mood disorder; samples followed up longitudinally appear to have more specific problems with antisocial behavior and substance abuse compared with healthy control subjects (Harrington et al. 1991; Weissman et al. 1999b). Adolescent onset of depression is more specifically associated with continuing problems with mood disorders in adulthood and less closely linked with antisocial behavior and other psychiatric outcomes (Harrington et al. 1990; Lewinsohn et al. 1999; Weissman et al. 1999a).

Course of a Mood Episode

The course of the mood episode in a given child is somewhat dependent on the chronicity and severity of the episode at presentation. Chronic forms of depressive illness have been reported in both community and clinical samples of children and adolescents (Goodman et al. 2000; Kovacs et al. 1994), and the chronicity of the index episode (determined at assessment) predicts both degree of impairment at presentation and, prospectively, the duration of the symptomatic impairment. For example, as with adults, if a child or an adolescent is given a chronic mood disorder diagnosis (such as dysthymic disorder) at presentation, the ensuing duration of symptomatic impairment can be as long as several years (Kovacs et al. 1994). More acute presentations of major depression may be more severe in their initial presentation but tend to resolve more quickly. The vast majority of mood episodes pre-

senting in youths will resolve over an ensuing prospective follow-up period if the child is followed up for a few years, and only
a small, unfortunate minority have essentially chronic, unremit-
ting symptoms of depression for as long as 5 years. However,
early onset of mood episodes in adolescence tends to predict recurrent mood episodes. In addition, depressed youths appear to
be at relatively high risk for developing future episodes of mania
or hypomania when followed up prospectively for several years
(Geller et al. 2001; Kovacs et al. 1994).

Long-Term Sequelae

Longitudinal follow-up of both clinical and community samples
of depressed youths shows serious morbidity associated with the
illness. Depressive illness diagnosed in children or adolescents
has been associated with future educational problems, peer relationship problems, negative self-image, the onset of substance
abuse, greater family conflict, suicide attempts, antisocial behavior, and psychiatric hospitalization (Harrington et al. 1991, 1994;
Lewinsohn et al. 1999; Weissman et al. 1999a, 1999b). In addition,
evidence suggests that the diagnosis of depression in youths,
even after personality traits present during childhood are controlled for, may predict the onset of personality disorder in later
adolescence or adulthood (Kasen et al. 2001).

Mortality

In addition to problems with suicidal ideation and nonlethal suicide attempts, depressive illness, especially in adolescents, has
been linked to death from suicide. Data supporting this association
have been derived primarily through two types of research studies. First, psychological autopsy studies from several research
groups concurred that depression, compared with other types of
psychiatric disorders, is a leading risk factor for completed suicide
in this age group, as is the case in adults (Brent et al. 1993b; Shaffer
et al. 1996b). Second, a recent longitudinal follow-up study of a
clinical sample of depressed adolescents reported a completed suicide rate of nearly 8% from the original sample, a strikingly higher
rate than found in the general population as well as in a non-

depressed comparison group, in which no one committed suicide (Weissman et al. 1999a). The vast majority of depressed youths do not commit suicide, but these studies do serve as reminders that depressive illness in youths is associated with a risk for mortality as well as significant morbidity.

References

Ambrosini PJ: Historical development and present status of the Schedule for Affective Disorders and Schizophrenia for School-Aged Children (K-SADS). J Am Acad Child Adolesc Psychiatry 39:49–58, 2000

Ambrosini PJ, Metz C, Bianchi MD, et al: Concurrent validity and psychometric properties of the Beck Depression Inventory in outpatient adolescents. J Am Acad Child Adolesc Psychiatry 30:51–57, 1991

American Psychiatric Association: Diagnostic and Statistical Manual of Mental Disorders, 3rd Edition. Washington, DC, American Psychiatric Association, 1980

American Psychiatric Association: Diagnostic and Statistical Manual of Mental Disorders, 4th Edition, Text Revision. Washington, DC, American Psychiatric Association, 2000

Andrews VC, Garrison CZ, Jackson KL, et al: Mother-adolescent agreement on the symptoms and diagnoses of adolescent depression and conduct disorders. J Am Acad Child Adolesc Psychiatry 32:731–738, 1993

Angold A, Costello EJ: The Child and Adolescent Psychiatric Assessment (CAPA). J Am Acad Child Adolesc Psychiatry 39:39–48, 2000

Angold A, Weissman MM, John K, et al: Parent and child reports of depressive symptoms in children at low and high risk of depression. J Child Psychol Psychiatry 28:901–915, 1987

Angold A, Costello EJ, Erkanli A, et al: Pubertal changes in hormone levels and depression in girls. Psychol Med 29:1043–1053, 1999

Beck AT, Ward CH, Mendelson H, et al: An inventory for measuring depression. Arch Gen Psychiatry 4:561–571, 1961

Biederman J, Rosenbaum JF, Bolduc-Murphy EA, et al: A 3-year follow-up of children with and without behavioral inhibition. J Am Acad Child Adolesc Psychiatry 32:814–821, 1993

Bird HR, Gould MS, Staghezza B: Aggregating data from multiple informants in child psychiatry epidemiological research. J Am Acad Child Adolesc Psychiatry 31:78–85, 1992

Bird HR, Gould MS, Staghezza BM: Patterns of diagnostic comorbidity in a community sample of children aged 9 through 16 years. J Am Acad Child Adolesc Psychiatry 32:361–368, 1993

Birmaher B, Dahl RE, Ryan ND, et al: The dexamethasone suppression test in adolescent outpatients with major depressive disorder. Am J Psychiatry 149:1040–1045, 1992a

Birmaher B, Ryan ND, Dahl R, et al: Dexamethasone suppression test in children with major depressive disorder. J Am Acad Child Adolesc Psychiatry 31:291–297, 1992b

Birmaher B, Kaufman J, Brent DA, et al: Neuroendocrine response to 5-hydroxy-L-tryptophan in prepubertal children at high risk of major depressive disorder. Arch Gen Psychiatry 54:1113–1119, 1997

Birmaher B, Dahl RE, Williamson DE, et al: Growth hormone secretion in children and adolescents at high risk for major depressive disorder. Arch Gen Psychiatry 57:867–872, 2000

Bonte FJ, Trivedi MH, Devous MDS, et al: Occipital brain perfusion deficits in children with major depressive disorder. J Nucl Med 42:1059–1061, 2001

Brent DA, Crumrine PK, Varma R, et al: Phenobarbital treatment and major depressive disorder in children with epilepsy: a naturalistic follow-up. Pediatrics 85:1086–1091, 1990

Brent DA, Perper JA, Moritz G, et al: Psychiatric impact of the loss of an adolescent sibling to suicide. J Affect Disord 28:249–256, 1993a

Brent DA, Perper JA, Moritz G, et al: Psychiatric risk factors for adolescent suicide: a case-control study. J Am Acad Child Adolesc Psychiatry 32:521–529, 1993b

Brent DA, Perper JA, Moritz G, et al: Psychiatric sequelae to the loss of an adolescent peer to suicide. J Am Acad Child Adolesc Psychiatry 32:509–517, 1993c

Cerel J, Fristad MA, Weller EB, et al: Suicide-bereaved children and adolescents: a controlled longitudinal examination. J Am Acad Child Adolesc Psychiatry 38:672–679, 1999

Cohen P, Cohen J, Kasen S, et al: An epidemiological study of disorders in late childhood and adolescence—I: age- and gender-specific prevalence. J Child Psychol Psychiatry 34:851–867, 1993

Cole DA: Relation of social and academic competence to depressive symptoms in childhood. J Abnorm Psychol 99:422–429, 1990

Costello EJ, Angold A, Burns BJ, et al: The Great Smoky Mountains Study of Youth: goals, design, methods, and the prevalence of DSM-III-R disorders. Arch Gen Psychiatry 53:1129–1136, 1996

Costello EJ, Erkanli A, Federman E, et al: Development of psychiatric comorbidity with substance abuse in adolescents: effects of timing and sex. J Clin Child Psychol 28:298–311, 1999

Cyranowski JM, Frank E, Young E, et al: Adolescent onset of the gender difference in lifetime rates of major depression: a theoretical model. Arch Gen Psychiatry 57:21–27, 2000

Cytryn L, McKnew DHJ: Proposed classification of childhood depression. Am J Psychiatry 129:63–69, 1972

Cytryn L, McKnew DHJ, Bunney WE Jr: Diagnosis of depression in children: a reassessment. Am J Psychiatry 137:22–25, 1980

Dahl RE: Sleep disorders, in Textbook of Pediatric Neuropsychiatry. Edited by Coffey CE, Brumback RA. Washington, DC, American Psychiatric Press, 1998, pp 821–838

Dorn LD, Dahl RE, Birmaher B, et al: Baseline thyroid hormones in depressed and non-depressed pre- and early pubertal boys and girls. J Psychiatr Res 31:555–567, 1997

Eaves LJ, Silberg JL, Meyer JM, et al: Genetics and developmental psychopathology, 2: the main effects of genes and environment on behavioral problems in the Virginia Twin Study of Adolescent Behavioral Development. J Child Psychol Psychiatry 38:965–980, 1997

Emslie GJ, Weinberg WA, Rush AJ, et al: Depression and dexamethasone suppression testing in children and adolescents. J Child Neurol 2:31–37, 1987

Emslie GJ, Rush AJ, Weinberg WA, et al: Children with major depression show reduced rapid eye movement latencies. Arch Gen Psychiatry 47:119–124, 1990

Emslie GJ, Rush AJ, Weinberg WA, et al: Sleep EEG features of adolescents with major depression. Biol Psychiatry 36:573–581, 1994

Emslie GJ, Armitage R, Weinberg WA, et al: Sleep polysomnography as a predictor of recurrence in children and adolescents with major depressive disorder. International Journal of Neuropsychopharmacology 4:159–168, 2001

Fergusson DM, Horwood LJ, Lynskey MT: Prevalence and comorbidity of DSM-III diagnoses in a birth cohort of 15 year olds. J Am Acad Child Adolesc Psychiatry 32:1127–1134, 1993

Fergusson DM, Horwood LJ, Beautrais AL: Is sexual orientation related to mental health problems and suicidality in young people? Arch Gen Psychiatry 56:876–880, 1999

Ferro T, Verdeli H, Pierre F, et al: Screening for depression in mothers bringing their offspring for evaluation or treatment of depression. Am J Psychiatry 157:375–379, 2000

Fleming JE, Offord DR, Boyle MH: Prevalence of childhood and adolescent depression in the community. Ontario Child Health Study. Br J Psychiatry 155:647–654, 1989

Garcia MR, Ryan ND, Rabinovitch H, et al: Thyroid stimulating hormone response to thyrotropin in prepubertal depression. J Am Acad Child Adolesc Psychiatry 30:398–406, 1991

Garland AF, Hough RL, McCabe KM, et al: Prevalence of psychiatric disorders in youths across five sectors of care. J Am Acad Child Adolesc Psychiatry 40:409–418, 2001

Garrison CZ, Addy CL, Jackson KL, et al: The CES-D as a screen for depression and other psychiatric disorders in adolescents. J Am Acad Child Adolesc Psychiatry 30:636–641, 1991

Garrison CZ, Addy CL, Jackson KL, et al: Major depressive disorder and dysthymia in young adolescents. Am J Epidemiol 135:792–802, 1992

Garrison CZ, Waller JL, Cuffe SP, et al: Incidence of major depressive disorder and dysthymia in young adolescents. J Am Acad Child Adolesc Psychiatry 36:458–465, 1997

Geller B, Zimerman B, Williams M, et al: Bipolar disorder at prospective follow-up of adults who had prepubertal major depressive disorder. Am J Psychiatry 158:125–127, 2001

Ghaziuddin N, King CA, Welch KB, et al: Serotonin dysregulation in adolescents with major depression: hormone response to meta-chlorophenylpiperazine (mCPP) infusion. Psychiatry Res 95:183–194, 2000

Goetz RR, Puig-Antich J, Ryan N, et al: Electroencephalographic sleep of adolescents with major depression and normal controls. Arch Gen Psychiatry 44:61–68, 1987

Goldston DB, Kovacs M, Ho VY, et al: Suicidal ideation and suicide attempts among youth with insulin-dependent diabetes mellitus. J Am Acad Child Adolesc Psychiatry 33:240–246, 1994

Goodman SH, Schwab-Stone M, Lahey BB, et al: Major depression and dysthymia in children and adolescents: discriminant validity and differential consequences in a community sample. J Am Acad Child Adolesc Psychiatry 39:761–770, 2000

Gotlib IH, Abramson LY: Attributional theories of emotion, in Handbook of Cognition and Emotion. Edited by Dalgleish T, Power M. West Sussex, England, Wiley, 1999, pp 613–636

Gould MS, King R, Greenwald S, et al: Psychopathology associated with suicidal ideation and attempts among children and adolescents. J Am Acad Child Adolesc Psychiatry 37:915–923, 1998

Hamilton M: Development of a rating for primary depressive illness. The British Journal of Social and Clinical Psychology 6:278–296, 1967

Hammen C, Rudolph K, Weisz J, et al: The context of depression in clinic-referred youth: neglected areas in treatment. J Am Acad Child Adolesc Psychiatry 38:64–71, 1999

Harrington R, Fudge H, Rutter M, et al: Adult outcomes of childhood and adolescent depression, I: psychiatric status. Arch Gen Psychiatry 47:465–473, 1990

Harrington R, Fudge H, Rutter M, et al: Adult outcomes of childhood and adolescent depression, II: links with antisocial disorders. J Am Acad Child Adolesc Psychiatry 30:434–439, 1991

Harrington R, Bredenkamp D, Groothues C, et al: Adult outcomes of childhood and adolescent depression, III: links with suicidal behaviours. J Child Psychol Psychiatry 35:1309–1319, 1994

Hughes CW, Petty F, Sheikha S, et al: Whole-blood serotonin in children and adolescents with mood and behavior disorders. Psychiatry Res 65:79–95, 1996

Hull PR, Demkiw-Bartel C: Isotretinoin use in acne: prospective evaluation of adverse events. J Cutan Med Surg 4:66–70, 2000

Johnson JG, Cohen P, Kasen S, et al: Association of maladaptive parental behavior with psychiatric disorder among parents and their offspring. Arch Gen Psychiatry 58:453–460, 2001

Kandel DB, Johnson JG, Bird HR, et al: Psychiatric comorbidity among adolescents with substance use disorders: findings from the MECA Study. J Am Acad Child Adolesc Psychiatry 38:693–699, 1999

Kasen S, Cohen P, Skodol AE, et al: Childhood depression and adult personality disorder: alternative pathways of continuity. Arch Gen Psychiatry 58:231–236, 2001

Kaufman J: Depressive disorders in maltreated children. J Am Acad Child Adolesc Psychiatry 30:257–265, 1991

King NJ, Bernstein GA: School refusal in children and adolescents: a review of the past 10 years. J Am Acad Child Adolesc Psychiatry 40:197–205, 2001

Klein DN, Lewinsohn PM, Seeley JR, et al: A family study of major depressive disorder in a community sample of adolescents. Arch Gen Psychiatry 58:13–20, 2001

Kovacs M: Rating scales to assess depression in school-aged children. Acta Paedopsychiatrica 46:305–315, 1981

Kovacs M: Presentation and course of major depressive disorder during childhood and later years of the life span. J Am Acad Child Adolesc Psychiatry 35:705–715, 1996

Kovacs M, Akiskal HS, Gatsonis C, et al: Childhood-onset dysthymic disorder: clinical features and prospective naturalistic outcome. Arch Gen Psychiatry 51:365–374, 1994

Kovacs M, Devlin B, Pollock M, et al: A controlled family history study of childhood-onset depressive disorder. Arch Gen Psychiatry 54:613–623, 1997

Kowatch RA, Devous MDS, Harvey DC, et al: A SPECT HMPAO study of regional cerebral blood flow in depressed adolescents and normal controls. Prog Neuropsychopharmacol Biol Psychiatry 23:643–656, 1999

Lewinsohn PM, Hops H, Roberts RE, et al: Adolescent psychopathology, I: prevalence and incidence of depression and other DSM-III-R disorders in high school students. J Abnorm Psychol 102:133–144, 1993

Lewinsohn PM, Rohde P, Seeley JR: Adolescent psychopathology, III: the clinical consequences of comorbidity. J Am Acad Child Adolesc Psychiatry 34:510–519, 1995

Lewinsohn PM, Rohde P, Seeley JR: Major depressive disorder in older adolescents: prevalence, risk factors, and clinical implications. Clin Psychol Rev 18:765–794, 1998

Lewinsohn PM, Rohde P, Klein DN, et al: Natural course of adolescent major depressive disorder, I: continuity into young adulthood. J Am Acad Child Adolesc Psychiatry 38:56–63, 1999

Lewinsohn PM, Solomon A, Seeley JR, et al: Clinical implications of "subthreshold" depressive symptoms. J Abnorm Psychol 109:345–351, 2000

Lewinsohn PM, Joiner TEJ, Rohde P: Evaluation of cognitive diathesis-stress models in predicting major depressive disorder in adolescents. J Abnorm Psychol 110:203–215, 2001

McClellan JM, Werry JS: Introduction—research psychiatric diagnostic interviews for children and adolescents. J Am Acad Child Adolesc Psychiatry 39:19–27, 2000

McGee R, Feehan M, Williams S, et al: DSM-III disorders in a large sample of adolescents. J Am Acad Child Adolesc Psychiatry 29:611–619, 1990

Monroe SM, Rohde P, Seeley JR, et al: Life events and depression in adolescence: relationship loss as a prospective risk factor for first onset of major depressive disorder. J Abnorm Psychol 108:606–614, 1999

Poznanski EO, Cook SC, Carroll BJ: A depression rating scale for children. Pediatrics 64:442–450, 1979

Puig-Antich J, Weston B: The diagnosis and treatment of major depressive disorder in childhood. Annu Rev Med 34:231–245, 1983

Puig-Antich J, Goetz R, Hanlon C, et al: Sleep architecture and REM sleep measures in prepubertal children with major depression: a controlled study. Arch Gen Psychiatry 39:932–939, 1982

Puig-Antich J, Goetz D, Davies M, et al: A controlled family history study of prepubertal major depressive disorder. Arch Gen Psychiatry 46:406–418, 1989

Reich W: Diagnostic Interview for Children and Adolescents (DICA). J Am Acad Child Adolesc Psychiatry 39:59–66, 2000

Renouf AG, Kovacs M: Concordance between mothers' reports and children's self-reports of depressive symptoms: a longitudinal study. J Am Acad Child Adolesc Psychiatry 33:208–216, 1994

Reynolds WM: Reliability and validity of the Reynolds Adolescent Depression Scale with young adolescents. Journal of School Psychology 36:295–312, 1998

Robins E, Guze SB: Establishment of diagnostic validity in psychiatric illness: its application to schizophrenia. Am J Psychiatry 126:983–987, 1970

Roosa MW, Reinholtz C, Angelini PJ: The relation of child sexual abuse and depression in young women: comparisons across four ethnic groups. J Abnorm Child Psychol 27:65–76, 1999

Ryan ND, Puig-Antich J, Ambrosini P, et al: The clinical picture of major depression in children and adolescents. Arch Gen Psychiatry 44:854–861, 1987

Ryan ND, Birmaher B, Perel JM, et al: Neuroendocrine response to L-5-hydroxytryptophan challenge in prepubertal major depression: depressed vs normal children. Arch Gen Psychiatry 49:843–851, 1992

Ryan ND, Dahl RE, Birmaher B, et al: Stimulatory tests of growth hormone secretion in prepubertal major depression: depressed versus normal children. J Am Acad Child Adolesc Psychiatry 33:824–833, 1994

Sallee FR, Hilal R, Dougherty D, et al: Platelet serotonin transporter in depressed children and adolescents: 3H-paroxetine platelet binding before and after sertraline. J Am Acad Child Adolesc Psychiatry 37:777–784, 1998

Seligman ME: Attributional style and depressive symptoms among children. J Abnorm Psychol 93:235–238, 1984

Shaffer D, Fisher P, Dulcan MK, et al: The NIMH Diagnostic Interview Schedule for Children Version 2.3 (DISC-2.3): description, acceptability, prevalence rates, and performance in the MECA Study. Methods for the Epidemiology of Child and Adolescent Mental Disorders Study. J Am Acad Child Adolesc Psychiatry 35:865–877, 1996a

Shaffer D, Gould MS, Fisher P, et al: Psychiatric diagnosis in child and adolescent suicide. Arch Gen Psychiatry 53:339–348, 1996b

Shaffer D, Fisher P, Lucas CP, et al: NIMH Diagnostic Interview Schedule for Children Version IV (NIMH DISC-IV): description, differences from previous versions, and reliability of some common diagnoses. J Am Acad Child Adolesc Psychiatry 39:28–38, 2000

Sheeber L, Allen N, Davis B, et al: Regulation of negative affect during mother-child problem-solving interactions: adolescent depressive status and family processes. J Abnorm Child Psychol 28:467–479, 2000

Sherrill JT, Kovacs M: Interview Schedule for Children and Adolescents (ISCA). J Am Acad Child Adolesc Psychiatry 39:67–75, 2000

Steingard RJ, Renshaw PF, Yurgelun-Todd D, et al: Structural abnormalities in brain magnetic resonance images of depressed children. J Am Acad Child Adolesc Psychiatry 35:307–311, 1996

Steingard RJ, Yurgelun-Todd DA, Hennen J, et al: Increased orbitofrontal cortex levels of choline in depressed adolescents as detected by in vivo proton magnetic resonance spectroscopy. Biol Psychiatry 48: 1053–1061, 2000

Weissman MM, Warner V, Wickramaratne P, et al: Offspring of depressed parents: 10 years later. Arch Gen Psychiatry 54:932–940, 1997

Weissman MM, Wolk S, Goldstein RB, et al: Depressed adolescents grown up. JAMA 281:1707–1713, 1999a

Weissman MM, Wolk S, Wickramarante P, et al: Children with prepubertal-onset major depressive disorder and anxiety grown up. Arch Gen Psychiatry 56:794–801, 1999b

Weller EB, Weller RA, Fristad MA, et al: The dexamethasone suppression test in prepubertal depressed children. J Clin Psychiatry 46:511–513, 1985

Weller EB, Weller RA, Fristad MA, et al: Children's Interview for Psychiatric Syndromes (ChIPS). J Am Acad Child Adolesc Psychiatry 39: 76–84, 2000

Whitaker A, Johnson J, Shaffer D, et al: Uncommon troubles in young people: prevalence estimates of selected psychiatric disorders in a nonreferred adolescent population. Arch Gen Psychiatry 47:487–496, 1990

Chapter 2

Psychotherapy for Depression and Suicidal Behavior in Children and Adolescents

Laura Mufson, Ph.D.
Drew M. Velting, Ph.D.

Only in the last decade has there been a significant initiative in the conduct of psychotherapy efficacy studies with depressed children and adolescents despite high prevalence and morbidity rates in this population. The intervention research literature on child and adolescent depression and suicide lags behind others that describe efficacy studies of adult and other childhood disorders. In this chapter, we provide a review of the major clinical trial studies evaluating outpatient psychotherapy for depressed children and adolescents as well as psychotherapy for suicidal youth. Only randomized controlled clinical trials targeting depressed youth are included to limit the review to studies most closely meeting criteria for empirically supported treatments. Because of the paucity of clinical trial research targeting suicidal behavior in youth, studies of varying designs are discussed.

Psychotherapeutic Interventions for Depressed Children and Adolescents

Background

Studies of Psychosocial Interventions

The literature describing psychosocial interventions for depressed youth has included many case studies and small single-subject designs. Until recently, scientifically rigorous randomized controlled clinical outcome studies were lacking. Most of the recent clinical trials investigated the efficacy of cognitive-behavioral treatments, with a smaller number examining interpersonal psychotherapy. Clinical trials generally include children and adolescents with major depression and/or dysthymia. Many of these studies need replication because of several methodological limitations, including 1) small sample sizes, 2) inclusion of nonreferred versus referred children, 3) treatment of mild to moderate versus severe symptoms, and 4) treatment of depressive symptomatology versus criterion-based diagnosis (Kovacs 1997). The studies we review are discussed in the context of these issues. We also review depression prevention studies that target "at risk" children based on elevated levels of self-reported depressive symptoms. We have excluded prevention studies targeting child offspring of depressed parents as well as universal prevention programs. Also, note that we focus on interpersonal psychotherapy and cognitive-behavioral therapy (CBT).

No randomized controlled clinical trials of a psychodynamic/psychoanalytic approach to treating depressed youth are currently available, in part because of the absence of treatment manuals, a necessary ingredient for conducting controlled trials. In addition, no controlled trials of family therapy for depressed youth have been published, although several models are currently under investigation (Diamond and Siqueland 1995; Fristad et al. 1998).

Empirically Based Treatment

Guidelines set forth by the Task Force on Promotion and Dissemination of Psychological Procedures (1996) propose several conditions that must be met for a treatment to be considered efficacious: 1) the treatment must be manual-based, 2) sample characteristics must be detailed, and 3) at least two different investigatory teams must show intervention effects (Kaslow and Thompson 1998). Kaslow and Thompson (1998) outlined the criteria that differentiate between "probably efficacious" and "well-established" treatments and concluded that only one treatment, The Coping With Depression Course (Lewinsohn et al. 1984)—Adolescent Adaptation, is close to meeting well-established criteria (Lewinsohn et al. 1996). The remainder of the studies are characterized by small sample sizes, testing only by the investigator who developed the treatment, and lack of comparison with another already established treatment. This last criterion is difficult to achieve because few efficacious treatments for youth depression are available to use as a basis for comparison. These intervention studies are also limited by the fact that most treatment approaches in use are downward extensions of adult treatment modalities (Mueller and Orvaschel 1997) and may not be developmentally appropriate.

The selection of an appropriate control group for a psychosocial treatment is a complicated issue and represents a key methodological challenge in clinical trials research. Discussion has focused on what constitutes the equivalent of a drug placebo for psychotherapy and ethical wait-list conditions if the former condition is not feasible to implement. Initially, researchers simply used a wait-list control condition, which meant that subjects received assessments without any therapy contact. Use of such a comparison group limits the extent to which findings can indicate that a treatment is superior to no treatment. To address the issue of whether techniques specific to a particular treatment model were the active ingredient rather than the nonspecific factors of treatment, researchers used the attention control condition as a comparison group. The attention control condition usually is characterized by meetings with a therapist who has been given strict instructions not to give advice or use any of the active therapeutic techniques being used in the treatment of interest for the study. More recently, the use of a treatment-as-usual comparison group has gained acceptance in the shift from conducting strict efficacy studies to conducting more effectiveness studies. Inclusion of this comparison group allows researchers to determine whether the specific modality being studied is superior to treatment usually delivered in that setting. However, treatment-as-usual may be hard to characterize, making it difficult to explain how it differs from the experimental treatment. These treatments must be differentiated to interpret the efficacy data and to attribute the effect to something unique in the experimental treatment. The field of psychosocial research continues to struggle with the notion of a "psychosocial placebo" and appropriate control conditions for an experimental psychotherapy condition.

The chapter is organized initially according to treatment models for depressed youth: CBT and interpersonal psychotherapy. Within each of these modalities, we review childhood and adolescent intervention studies. We then review prevention studies conducted with at-risk children and adolescents. These discussions are followed by a review of approaches to the treatment of suicidal youth.

Cognitive-Behavioral Therapy Model of Depression

CBT is based on the premise that negative thinking contributes to the development and maintenance of depressive symptoms (Beck et al. 1979). The model assumes that negative thinking leads to negative affect states and maladaptive behaviors. Negative automatic thoughts and core beliefs are targeted as "hypotheses" that can be evaluated empirically, based on personal observation and self-monitoring. Patients also learn how to make connections between cognitions and depressed affect, to alter these beliefs, and to use adaptive problem-solving skills (Emery et al. 1983). Cognitive distortions have been identified as a risk factor for the development of depressive symptomatology in children and adolescents (Garber et al. 1993).

The behavioral component of CBT has its roots in reinforcement theory. According to Lewinsohn et al. (1969), depressed individuals do not have access to sufficient schedules of positive reinforcement because of either access problems or skill deficits.

An increase in pleasurable activities is associated with a decrease in depressive symptomatology (Lewinsohn et al. 1996). Ways to increase pleasurable activities, problem-solving skills, social skills and assertiveness training, and emotion regulation techniques are taught. The goal is to increase positive reinforcement from the activities directly and from improved interpersonal relationships that may be a secondary outcome of the activities. Several different CBT manuals have been developed, but they all share the same basic theoretical foundation.

Child Intervention Studies

Currently, there are at least 13 randomized controlled clinical trials of CBT with depressed youth (Harrington 1998b). The studies vary according to referral source (advertisement, pediatrician, mental health clinic, or school), treatment setting, selection of control conditions, and whether children meet criteria for a DSM disorder or report symptoms of a subsyndromal nature.

Symptomatic community samples.   Most treatment studies with depressed children were actually conducted on site in schools and included children with depressive symptoms but who did not necessarily meet criteria for a disorder (Butler et al. 1980; Kahn et al. 1990; Liddle and Spence 1990; Stark et al. 1987; Weisz et al. 1997). Participants usually are screened with a self-report instrument such as the Children's Depression Inventory (CDI; Kovacs 1985) and are recruited within the schools. Typical cutoff scores of 13 or greater on the CDI or 40 or greater on the Children's Depression Rating Scale, Revised (CDRS-R; Poznanski and Mokros 1996), suggest clinically significant levels of depression. Formal diagnoses are not made because information about duration and frequency of symptoms is lacking. These instruments often are used as outcome measures along with a measure of self-esteem. The designs of the studies are generally similar in that CBT is most often compared with another active treatment and a wait-list control. In these studies, CBT is typically brief (25 sessions or fewer) and delivered in a group format at the end of the regular school day.

Several studies have compared CBT with attention placebo or

wait-list conditions delivered in a school setting (Butler et al. 1980; Kahn et al. 1990; Liddle and Spence 1990; Weisz et al. 1997). The studies generally included children from third to sixth grade who were found to have elevated levels of depressive symptoms on a grade- or schoolwide screening. Collectively, findings indicated that children treated with some form of CBT showed greater reduction in depressive symptoms than did those who received either attention placebo (Butler et al. 1980) or a wait-list condition (Kahn et al. 1990; Weisz et al. 1997). Weisz et al. (1997) reported that primary and secondary enhancement training was effective and that the effects were maintained at 9-month follow-up. Kahn et al. (1990) also reported greater reductions in depressive symptoms for children treated with CBT, relaxation training, and a self-modeling intervention than for those in the wait-list condition at the conclusion of the acute phase and at 1-month follow-up.

The exception to these findings was the Liddle and Spence (1990) study, which reported no differences between social competence training, attention placebo control, and a no-treatment control condition in regard to reduction of depressive symptoms or improving social competence posttreatment and at 3-month follow-up. All subjects ($N=32$) reported a decline in depression scores during the treatment period. This discrepancy in findings may be a result of the inclusion of younger patients (7- and 8-year-olds), who may have been too cognitively immature to take full advantage of the social competence training, and the small sample size for the three treatment conditions.

Stark et al. (1987) compared two types of group therapy (self-control therapy and behavioral problem-solving therapy) in treating 29 children (fourth to sixth graders) with depressive symptoms labeled as dysphoria. The children were randomly assigned to self-control therapy, behavioral problem-solving therapy, or wait-list condition. Treatment was delivered in twelve 50-minute sessions over a 5-week period. The children in the two active treatments reported significantly greater reduction in depressive symptoms than did those on the wait list; however, outcomes for the two active treatments were comparable. A follow-up study showed that the children were able to maintain these gains at

8 weeks after acute treatment. In a second study, Stark et al. (1991) randomly assigned 24 fourth to seventh graders with elevated depressive symptoms to either 24–26 sessions of cognitive-behavioral self-control therapy with monthly family meetings or traditional counseling. They found that the children in both groups showed a reduction in depressive symptoms posttreatment and at 7-month follow-up, with some increased advantage for the CBT, although the difference was not statistically significant. The results were limited by the small sample size.

With the exception of the study by Liddle and Spence (1990), these studies suggested that for the preadolescent age group, CBT is not superior to other active treatments in reducing depressive symptoms, although it is superior to maintaining children on a wait list. Active treatments tend to result in superior effects relative to wait-list control, but CBT does not produce responses significantly different from those of relaxation training or traditional counseling (Kahn et al. 1990; Stark et al. 1991). The similarity in results of the active treatments (Butler et al. 1980; Stark et al. 1987) may be accounted for by the fact that they appear to be variations of CBT albeit with emphases on different techniques.

Clinically referred samples. No current studies are available on the use of CBT in a clinically referred sample of prepubertal children.

Adolescent Intervention Studies

Early treatment efficacy studies for adolescents closely resembled those conducted with children. Reynolds and Coates (1986) reported on a clinical trial comparing CBT, relaxation training, and wait-list control for the treatment of elevated depressive symptoms in 30 adolescents. Group CBT was conducted in ten 50-minute meetings over 5 weeks. Like the studies with preadolescents, the two active treatments were superior to wait list in the reduction of depressive symptoms, with no differences identified between the two active treatments. The lack of difference between the two active treatments also could be due to the small sample size.

Fine et al. (1991) compared a social skills training group with a therapeutic support group, each consisting of five sessions over 12 weeks for 66 adolescents meeting DSM-III-R (American Psychiatric Association 1987) criteria for depression or dysthymia. Although not randomized in the strictest sense, the groups were run alternately, so adolescents were assigned to whichever treatment was being conducted at the time of their recruitment. Posttreatment, adolescents in the therapeutic support group showed significantly greater improvements in depression and self-concept compared with adolescents in the social skills training group. At 9-month follow-up, no group differences were seen because the therapeutic support group improvement was maintained, whereas the social skills group improved over time, suggesting delayed benefit for the social skills training program (Fine et al. 1991).

Community samples.   Lewinsohn et al. (1990) conducted a controlled clinical trial of group CBT (Coping With Depression Course) for 54 clinically depressed adolescents. Subjects were identified in school screenings, were diagnosed with the Schedule for Affective Disorders and Schizophrenia for School-Aged Children, Epidemiological Version (K-SADS-E), and met Research Diagnostic Criteria for major, minor, and intermittent depression. The Coping With Depression Course consists of fourteen 2-hour sessions over 7 weeks conducted on site after school. Adolescents received the Coping With Depression Course either with or without seven parent group sessions, and the two active treatment conditions were compared with adolescents in a wait-list control condition. Adolescents in the two group CBT conditions improved significantly more on depressive measures than did subjects assigned to the wait-list control condition. No significant difference was found between adolescents whose parents did and did not participate in the treatment program, although a trend suggested that parental involvement may provide increased benefits for the reduction of depressive symptoms (Lewinsohn et al. 1990). The parental component may prove to be more beneficial for preadolescents who show greater dependency and for whom problems are more likely to be affected by the parental/familial context. The added benefit of parental involvement has yet to be empirically proven for the treatment of depression in adolescents.

Clarke et al. (1992) examined predictors of treatment outcome in the same sample and found that lower levels of depression and superior pretreatment psychosocial functioning (characterized by lower anxiety, higher enjoyment and frequency of pleasant activities, and more rational thoughts) at intake were strong predictors of reduction in depression symptoms at posttreatment. Lewinsohn et al. (1996) replicated the findings in a sample of 96 adolescents with major depression whose treatment was modified from the earlier trial by the inclusion of additional skills training and follow-up sessions. During the 2-year follow-up period, a third of the sample received booster sessions every 4 months for 2 years, another third was assessed every 4 months but received no booster sessions, and another third was assessed annually with no boosters. Adolescents who received the active treatments reported significant declines in depressive symptoms compared with the wait-list control group, but again there was no difference between Coping With Depression Course with and without parental involvement. At follow-up, no differences were found between the three follow-up conditions, indicating that booster sessions appeared to have little to no effect (Lewinsohn et al. 1996). This may be because of the relatively low number of booster sessions (three per year). The effectiveness may be augmented if booster sessions were more frequent, such as monthly.

Clarke et al. (1999) conducted another study examining the effectiveness of acute and maintenance Coping With Depression Course for 123 adolescents with major depression or dysthymic disorder. These adolescents differed from subjects in the earlier studies in that they were recruited not from schools but via announcements to mental health professionals and school counselors and television and newspaper advertising. The investigators replicated previous results. The difference between active and wait-list conditions was smaller than previously found because the rate of recovery for the wait-list condition increased, although the overall mean rate of recovery was higher (67%) in this trial than previously (46%) (Clarke et al. 1999). Although the boosters were intended to be studied in regard to their ability to prevent relapse in those who were recovered, the investigators randomized all subjects to either boosters or assessment only. Boosters did not significantly reduce the rate of recurrence in those adolescents already recovered at the end of the acute treatment but rather appeared to accelerate the rate of recovery for those adolescents who were still depressed at the end of the acute treatment phase. Attendance was estimated at less than 50%; consequently, the supplemental booster sessions were not optimally implemented. Given that the adolescents' rate of improvement was so high in the acute phase, motivation among the recovered to participate may have been low. The investigators suggested that the booster might better serve as a continuation treatment to help those not yet recovered at the end of the acute phase to achieve recovery faster during a post–acute phase of treatment (Clarke et al. 1999). This is conceptually distinct from a maintenance treatment, the goal of which is to maintain recovery and/or remission.

Clinical samples.   Wood et al. (1996) conducted a controlled clinical trial in which they compared brief individual CBT with relaxation training in clinically depressed adolescent outpatients. CBT was quite brief (five to eight sessions) and integrated techniques from a variety of treatment manuals that focused on changing cognitive distortions, interpersonal problem-solving skills training, and symptom-focused interventions. The integrated treatment was called the depression treatment program. Adolescents who received the depression treatment program reported significantly greater reduction in depression symptoms and improved overall functioning than did those in the relaxation condition. Remission was more likely at the end of the trial for the depression treatment program subjects (54%) than for those adolescents in the relaxation control condition (26%). At 6-month follow-up, no significant group differences were found; the relaxation group continued to report improvement in symptoms, whereas the depression treatment program group reported re-emergence of symptoms. Jayson et al. (1998) found that better outcome was associated with earlier diagnosis and higher baseline functioning in adolescents who had participated in two CBT studies (Kroll et al. 1996; Wood et al. 1996).

Vostanis et al. (1996a) compared the depression treatment program with what they called a nonfocused intervention, designed to be equivalent to an attention placebo condition. They found no significant group difference for recovery rates at the end of treatment and at 9-month follow-up. A high rate (46%) of the patients reported a depressive episode during the 9-month follow-up (Vostanis et al. 1996b).

One of the largest randomized controlled trials to date was conducted by Brent et al. (1997), who demonstrated the efficacy of individual CBT for depressed adolescents in comparison to structured behavioral family therapy and nondirective supportive psychotherapy in a clinically referred sample of 107 adolescents aged 13–18 years. CBT resulted in lower rates of major depressive disorder at the end of treatment and more rapid relief according to both interviewer ratings and patient report. All three treatments showed similar reductions in suicidality and functional impairments (Brent et al. 1997).

The adolescents were followed up for 2 years after completion of the acute trial to document the subsequent course of major depressive disorder (Birmaher et al. 2000). A portion of the adolescents received two to four booster sessions, and another received more extensive treatment for a variety of problems, including depression, behavior difficulties, and family conflicts. No significant differences in long-term outcome occurred among CBT, structured behavioral family therapy, and nondirective supportive psychotherapy conditions despite the superiority of CBT during the acute phase of treatment. A high proportion (80%) of the adolescents had recovered during the 2-year follow-up, whereas 30% reported a recurrence of depression during the follow-up period. The median time to remission from baseline was 5.7 months, and almost two-thirds of the remissions had occurred after the conclusion of the acute psychotherapy trial. This suggests that 16 weeks of psychotherapy may not be sufficient for most adolescents to achieve remission. The fact that 21% of the adolescents reported being depressed during at least 80% of the follow-up period (Birmaher et al. 2000) suggests that a large portion of the sample was severely and more chronically depressed. The lack of benefit for CBT over other treatments at follow-up is consistent with other studies (e.g., Wood et al. 1996). Functional or social role improvement occurred most often during the follow-up phase of the study. This is consistent with evidence indicating the persistence of social impairment beyond depressive symptom remission (Puig-Antich et al. 1993).

Lack of recovery and likelihood of recurrence were predicted by severity of depression at baseline, recruitment through a clinical setting versus advertisement, and self-reported parent-child conflict at baseline and during the follow-up period (Brent et al. 1998). Adolescents who had comorbid anxiety disorders and higher levels of cognitive distortion and hopelessness at intake were more likely to be depressed at the end of acute treatment. The efficacy of CBT significantly decreased in the presence of maternal depression, which is a common problem in families of depressed children. Ferro et al. (2000) are currently studying the extent to which treating depressed mothers affects the child's course of depression as an innovative approach to addressing this problem. In analyses controlling for the number of adverse predictors present, CBT continued to be the best of the three treatments and thus may be more likely to maintain its efficacy under real-world conditions that often are characterized by these adverse predictors (Brent et al. 1998).

Three meta-analyses of randomized controlled clinical trials involving CBT for depressed adolescents have been published (Harrington et al. 1998b; Lewinsohn and Clarke 1999; Reinecke et al. 1998). In reviewing six controlled trials in which CBT had most often been compared with a wait-list control, Harrington et al. (1998b) found that the rate of remission from depressive disorder was higher in the CBT group (62%) than in the comparison group (36%; odds ratio=3.2). Reinecke et al. (1998) cast a wider net and included 14 posttreatment control comparison studies of child and adolescent depression. They found an effect size of 1.02 for CBT at the conclusion of acute treatment. Lewinsohn and Clarke (1999) found an effect size of 1.27 for CBT and that 63% of the patients showed significant clinical improvement by the end of acute treatment. All of these authors concluded that reasonably good evidence supports the use of CBT to treat depression in children and adolescents; however, some room for improvement remains.

The high proportion of treated adolescents who fail to remit has been impetus for introducing the notion of a continuation and/or maintenance treatment. *Continuation treatment* refers to the continuation of therapy for several months after apparent partial or full remission at the end of acute treatment to ensure a complete remission and full recovery. *Maintenance treatment* refers to the continuation of therapy after full remission and recovery to prevent relapse and recurrence. Kroll et al. (1996) found that the addition of six monthly CBT booster sessions after the conclusion of acute treatment resulted in a much lower relapse rate (20%) than if children received acute CBT treatment only (50%). Research on prevention of recurrence through continuation or maintenance phase therapy is still in the early stages. Based on high recurrence rates, the American Academy of Child and Adolescent Psychiatry (1998) has incorporated continuation and maintenance treatment into its practice parameters for depression.

Prevention Studies

Children

Although results of these numerous CBT studies are encouraging, future efforts are needed to determine whether episodes can be prevented. Research on relapse prevention is just beginning with the initiation of more follow-up studies of children and adolescents who have participated in clinical trials. There is a similar movement to study whether children at risk for depression can be successfully identified and effectively treated to prevent future depressive episodes. However, primary prevention studies are complicated; participants must be studied over long periods to assess the preventive effect of the intervention.

The PENN Prevention Program was designed to prevent depressive symptoms among at-risk 10- to 13-year-old children. A 5-year prospective study assessed the effectiveness of three versions of the PENN Prevention Program—a cognitive training component, a social problem-solving component, and a combined treatment that included both components—compared with a wait-list control group and a no-participation control group. The latter two control groups were analyzed together as the control condition for the immediate and 6-month follow-up analyses. The goal was to target cognitive distortions and deficiencies in at-risk children, increase their sense of skill and mastery, and address problems such as lowered academic achievement, poor peer relationships, poor self-esteem, and some behavior problems (Jaycox et al. 1994). Children were identified as being at risk because of subsyndromal depressive symptoms and reports of parental conflict.

Subjects were recruited from the fifth and sixth grades, screened for depressive symptoms, and then given the opportunity to participate or not in the program. This type of recruitment may cause self-selection that may affect study results. The experimental conditions were assigned without bias to schools rather than to children (Jaycox et al. 1994). At posttreatment, depressive symptoms were significantly reduced and classroom behavior was significantly improved in the treatment group as compared with the control group. A 6-month follow-up showed continued reduction in depressive symptoms and conduct problems in comparison to control subjects. Children considered most at risk because of the number of target symptoms at baseline showed the greatest symptom reduction. perhaps because they had a greater range of potential improvement or had been more motivated to change. Given the absence of an attention control condition, it is not possible to rule out nonspecific treatment effects.

Children in the PENN Prevention Program were matched to a no-treatment control group and followed up for 2 years (Gilham et al. 1995). At follow-up, 44% of the children in the control group reported moderate to severe levels of depressive symptoms (CDI score≥15) in comparison to 22% in the PENN Prevention Program. Data from the Children's Attributional Style Questionnaire indicated that the PENN Prevention Program resulted in improvements in children's explanatory style characterized by an increase in optimistic statements. The change in explanatory style for negative events was found to be a mediator of the program's effect on depressive symptoms, and the prevention effect on depressive symptoms increased over time. Although the study had design limitations (lack of randomization, no attention control group, self-reported information), results suggested that cognitive interventions begun in late childhood might be effective in preventing future depression. The investigators are currently attempting to replicate this work with a randomized design.

Adolescents

Clarke et al. (1993) conducted two studies investigating school-based primary prevention of depressive symptoms in ninth- and tenth-grade adolescents. These first attempts at prevention showed little to no benefits. In 1995, Clarke and colleagues conducted another targeted prevention study of depression in an at-risk sample of high school adolescents. The adolescents were selected with a two-stage case-finding procedure. Those with an elevated Center for Epidemiologic Studies Depression Scale (CES-D) score ($\geq$24) on initial screening were interviewed with the K-SADS. Those subjects with current affective diagnoses were referred for other treatment. The remaining 150 consenting adolescents were considered at risk for future depression and randomized to receive either "usual care" or the Coping With Stress Course (a modification of the longer Coping With Depression Course) consisting of three 45-minute sessions per week for 5 weeks. The treatment goal was to teach new coping strategies that would provide the adolescent with some measure of protection or resistance against later development of depression (Clarke et al. 1995).

Over the 12-month follow-up period, adolescents in the Coping With Stress condition had a total incidence of unipolar depressive disorder that was approximately half that of the control group: 15% of the students who received the Coping With Stress Course reported a new episode of depression compared with 26% of the students in the control group. The onset of new episodes tended to occur within the first 2–3 months of the project, suggesting that some of the adolescents may have been identified in the prodromal period of a full depressive episode. This is the conundrum of prevention research. Is there a meaningful difference between being "demoralized" (Clarke et al. 1995) and being in a prodromal state of depression? It is an important question when determining how to correctly identify children and adolescents who are appropriate for preventive intervention. In the case of a prodromal state, greater effects might be achieved through active treatment intervention rather than with prevention alone.

Interpersonal Psychotherapy for Depressed Adolescents

Interpersonal psychotherapy for depressed adolescents (IPT-A) is an adaptation of IPT, a brief treatment originally developed for depressed, nonbipolar adults (Klerman et al. 1984). IPT places the depressive episode in the context of interpersonal relationships and focuses on current interpersonal conflicts. The goals of IPT are 1) to decrease depressive symptomatology and 2) to improve interpersonal functioning. IPT has been adapted to treat outpatient adolescents who have a nonbipolar, nonpsychotic depressive episode. Clinical research conducted in the 1970s and 1980s clearly established the efficacy of IPT for the treatment of nonbipolar depression in outpatient adults (DiMascio et al. 1979; Elkin et al. 1989; Weissman et al. 1979).

An interpersonal approach to the treatment of depression is well supported by research (Hammen 1999; Joiner et al. 1999). Researchers have found that depression, even at subclinical levels, is related to significant interpersonal problems and interpersonal stress (Aseltine et al. 1994; Puig-Antich et al. 1985, 1993; Stader and Hokanson 1998). Research has shown that interpersonal experiences are often precipitants of the onset of depression (Hammen 1999).

Adaptation for Depressed Adolescents

The treatment has been adapted to address developmental issues most common to adolescents, including separation from parents; development of dyadic, romantic interpersonal relationships; initial experiences with the death of a relative or friend; and peer pressures. Discussing interpersonal events is something many adolescents can relate to and are accustomed to in their daily lives. Strategies were developed for including family members in various phases of the treatment as needed. All of the modifications were organized into a treatment manual specifically designed for depressed adolescents (Mufson et al. 1993). To date, two controlled clinical trials of IPT for depressed adolescents have been published.

Mufson and colleagues (1994, 1999; Mufson and Fairbanks 1996) have been engaged in a programmatic study of IPT-A in a sample of minority, poor, urban, depressed adolescents. A controlled clinical trial of IPT-A for depressed adolescents in comparison to a clinical management control group (once a month supportive therapy) was conducted with a sample of 48 clinically referred adolescents with a diagnosis of major depressive disorder. Results showed that those adolescents who received IPT-A, as compared with clinical management, reported significantly greater reductions in depressive symptomatology and greater improvements in overall social functioning and certain social problem-solving skills. Specifically, they reported greater improvement in functioning with friends and in the ability to generate alternative solutions to problems as well as solution implementation and verification, as measured by the Social Problem Solving Inventory. Significantly more patients who received IPT-A (75%) as compared with control patients (46%) met recovery criteria for depression. Eighty-eight percent of the adolescents receiving IPT-A completed the 12-week protocol in comparison to 46% of the adolescents in the control condition.

In a study of 71 adolescents in Puerto Rico, Rossello and Bernal (1999) compared either CBT or IPT with wait list in subjects with major depressive disorder and/or dysthymia. This is one of only two studies (along with Brent et al. 1997) to compare two manualized active interventions. Pretreatment, posttreatment, and 3-month follow-up measures of depressive symptoms, self-esteem, social adjustment, family emotional involvement, criticism, and behavior problems were completed. Both IPT and CBT significantly reduced depressive symptoms in comparison to wait-list control, with IPT showing a little more benefit than CBT for improving general functioning. Depression recovery rates were 82% for IPT and 59% for CBT (Rossello and Bernal 1999).

Limitations of this study included attendance problems (68% IPT vs. 52% CBT) and concerns about criteria for recovery and its implications for comparison to other studies. The investigators did not assess diagnostic status posttreatment; rather, they reported a significant reduction in depressive symptoms by adolescent report. Despite the limitations, the two studies of IPT together suggest that it is an acceptable and efficacious treatment for adolescent depression in a specialty mental health setting.

Summary of Findings

Most studies of depressed youth focus on the efficacy of CBT rather than other therapeutic orientations. Preliminary evidence suggests that CBT has beneficial effects on recovery from depressive symptoms as well as from the disorder. Interestingly, CBT is not superior to other active treatments in prepubertal children, although it has been found to be superior for adolescents. Perhaps preadolescents are not cognitively mature enough to take full advantage of CBT as it now stands. These findings also may be due to power limitations from the consistently small sample sizes in the prepubertal studies. Further adaptation of CBT to more appropriately address cognitive level of development may be needed to improve its efficacy for the prepubertal population. In addition, further studies need to be conducted with prepubertal children meeting criteria for the disorder rather than dysphoria.

For adolescents, CBT is superior to a variety of therapies; however, a substantial number of adolescents still do not benefit, and the rate of recurrence after acute treatment is relatively high. In general, it appears that severely depressed adolescents respond less strongly to CBT than do adolescents with a mild to moderate severity of diagnosis (Brent et al. 1998). Follow-up periods for these studies rarely exceed a year, so the longer-term benefits of these treatments are still relatively unknown. Studies also show the promise of IPT as a treatment for depressed adolescents, but follow-up data are needed to assess its longer-term benefits. The generalizability of all these studies is limited by their inclusion of relatively homogenous samples with few comorbid diagnoses. These samples are not representative of the population in clinics and private offices. Once efficacy is suggested for a treatment, future studies should have less stringent exclusion criteria to more closely approximate those patients seen in real-world clinical settings.

Additional efforts are needed to further broaden the study of psychosocial treatments for depressed children and adolescents. Relatively few studies have compared two or more empirically supported active treatments for depressed youth. No published studies have compared psychotherapy with medication, although the National Institute of Mental Health (NIMH)–sponsored Treatment for Adolescents With Depression Study is under way. In addition, there are no large studies of empirically based treatments for the prevention of relapse in adolescents successfully treated for depression. Amid criticism of the restrictiveness of efficacy studies and concerns about the generalizability of the findings, alternative treatment models have been proposed that may incorporate more flexibility for therapists. These include designs for studying the sequencing of treatments (both psychosocial and pharmacological) to better address comorbid disorders that accompany depression. Also proposed are modular psychotherapy manuals that provide treatment algorithms that correspond to particular comorbidity profiles. For example, an adolescent with depression and posttraumatic stress disorder (PTSD) might receive IPT-A to treat the depression followed by another module providing more CBT-like treatment for the PTSD. As of yet, no studies have examined the efficacy of sequencing or modular treatments and the potential for greater generalizability of findings.

Several studies have begun to explore the notion of continuation treatment to increase the likelihood of achieving remission and to accelerate the recovery of adolescents who still report symptoms after the acute phase of treatment as well as maintenance treatment. The notion of preventing depression given its significant social morbidity is an exciting one but also one that is complicated by the need to identify for whom these programs would be most beneficial and to decide what is an acceptable follow-up period. Ideally, one would need to follow up children through adolescence into young adulthood to monitor them through the period of greatest risk for developing depression and know the full effect of the treatments. The two existing prevention studies provide support for pursuing the development of such programs targeting children at risk for depression through a variety of pathways. The goal is to give psychological "immunization" to children entering puberty that could serve to alleviate the serious public health consequences of adolescent depression (Gilham et al. 1995). Great inroads have been made in the treatment of depression, but a significant need for further study remains.

Despite the positive findings from many of these efficacy studies on depression, researchers and clinicians are unable to generalize the findings to more community-based settings in which clinical services are often delivered in less-than-optimal conditions, patient populations are more complex, and therapists' backgrounds and training are more varied. Recently, there has been increased emphasis on the importance of establishing not only the efficacy but also the effectiveness of treatments (Hoagwood et al. 1995). Effectiveness research is thought to better capture the effect of treatments on individuals who may have comorbid conditions and situations that might otherwise exclude them from more traditional efficacy studies. Mufson and several other researchers are currently conducting such effectiveness studies in settings such as primary care clinics and school-based health clinics. These studies should provide knowledge about treatment implementation and clinical effectiveness, as well as the cost-effectiveness of providing evidence-based treatments such as IPT for depressed adolescents and CBT in community settings.

Psychotherapeutic Treatments for Suicidal Children and Adolescents

In this section, we provide a critical review of *outpatient* psychotherapy interventions aimed at reducing suicidal ideation and behavior in youth. Such treatment is generally indicated as a follow-up to acute management of a suicidal episode, which often involves evaluation in an emergency service setting, crisis intervention, and, in some cases, inpatient or partial hospitalization. Thus, outpatient care is intended to supervene when the patient's condition has been stabilized and a reasonable degree of safety is assured (American Academy of Child and Adolescent Psychiatry 2001). Of course, this treatment "cycle" may be disrupted in instances when suicide risk cannot be managed effectively on an outpatient basis and acute care is again indicated. Although each of these stages is integral to a "wraparound" system of service delivery (Rotheram-Borus et al. 1996b), discussion of acute patient care in the context of suicidality is beyond the scope of this chapter.

Background

Whereas suicide among school-aged children (5- to 14-year-olds) is a relatively infrequent occurrence, adolescent suicide is now recognized as a major public health problem, accounting for nearly 2,000 deaths nationwide each year among 15- to 19-year-olds. Suicide is the third leading cause of death for this age group. Moreover, recent studies indicate that approximately 20% of the adolescents in community samples report serious suicidal ideation and between 3% and 8% report having made at least one suicide attempt (Centers for Disease Control and Prevention 2000). A range of risk factors has been identified for completed suicide (e.g., Brent et al. 1993; Gould et al. 1996; Shaffer et al. 1996) and nonlethal suicidal behavior in adolescents (e.g., Andrews and Lewinsohn 1992; Gould et al. 1998), but efficacious treatments for suicidal youth are not currently available. This highlights the need for the development and empirical validation of innovative psychotherapy interventions that specifically target risk factors such as depression, hopelessness, suicidal thoughts, and self-harm behaviors in clinically referred adolescents.

Drug therapy with selective serotonin reuptake inhibitors (SSRIs) such as fluoxetine has been suggested as a potentially effective treatment for suicidal adolescents with major depressive disorder (Greenhill and Waslick 1997), but at present, limited data are available. Because of concerns of safety and the lack of efficacy data, psychosocial treatment interventions provide a safe and effective alternative.

Limited Knowledge Base

Recent reviews of the treatment outcome literature (e.g., Rudd et al. 2000) note that few studies have systematically evaluated psychotherapy interventions aimed at reducing suicidal ideation and behavior in children and adolescents (i.e., randomized controlled trials that obtain reliable and valid measures of outcome variables during pretreatment, posttreatment, and follow-up periods). Reasonable explanations for this deficiency include the fact that most treatment efficacy studies of adolescent psychiatric populations exclude suicidal individuals from participation by design. High-risk youth with current suicidal ideation or a history of suicidal behavior often are excluded from clinical trials based on notions that potential risks outweigh benefits and that researchers are not adequately trained to handle suicidal crises (Pearson et al. 2001).

Challenges to Conducting Treatment Studies With Suicidal Youth

The conduct of suicide intervention research poses several unique challenges to investigators. Procedural complexity is considerable when suicidal patients are included in clinical trials. The NIMH recently published a paper (Pearson et al. 2001) that highlights some ethical, legal, and safety considerations associated with such studies. According to the NIMH, interventions designed to reduce suicidal ideation and behavior are considered high risk and therefore may require special research design modifications, enhanced safety monitoring procedures, and the establishment of well-defined risk management protocols. For example, investigators conducting clinical trials involving suicidal subjects are required to establish contingencies for managing and reporting adverse events (e.g., suicide attempts) that occur during treatment. Researchers in this area also must develop detailed risk management protocols that describe risk assessment procedures and specify decision rules for treatment planning and crisis intervention. Perceived liability risks also may deter investigators from the conduct of research with suicidal patients. The most common basis for litigation involving mental health professionals is the failure to prevent a patient's suicide (Gutheil 1999).

Generally low rates of treatment compliance among adolescent suicide attempters (e.g., Piacentini et al. 1995; Spirito et al. 1989) also make such investigations difficult to implement. Spirito et al. (1992) examined psychotherapy dropout rates for suicidal adolescents who were referred to treatment after inpatient hospitalization. At 3-month follow-up, only 59% of the adolescents in the sample had been regularly compliant with psychotherapy aftercare. Trautman et al. (1993) compared treatment compliance rates of adolescent suicide attempters referred for outpatient psychiatric care ($n=115$) with those of nonattempting adolescents who presented to the same clinical service ($n=110$). Survival analyses showed that the median number of sessions attended before dropout was 3 for attempters and 11 for nonattempters, demonstrating that attempters attended fewer sessions and showed more rapid rates of dropout. There is some indication that individual rather than family therapy is a more viable treatment option for suicidal adolescents. King et al. (1997) reported rates of treatment compliance for suicidal adolescents following hospitalization: 50.8% for individual therapy and 33.3% for family therapy/parent psychoeducation. Noncompliance with both modalities was generally associated with parental psychopathology and family dysfunction.

Some evidence suggests that implementation of specialized emergency room (ER) procedures may increase treatment adherence among Latina adolescent suicide attempters (Rotheram-Borus et al. 1996a, 1999). The procedures augmented typical ER care by 1) using a standardized protocol for training ER staff, 2) presenting a 20-minute videotape to patients and their families that modeled realistic expectations for aftercare treatment, and 3) providing a bilingual crisis therapist to promote compliance with outpatient therapy. Suicidal adolescents receiving the specialized ER procedure attended 3.8 more sessions than did those receiving standard aftercare, indicating that the specialized procedure was effective as a method for enhancing adolescent compliance.

Treatment Studies of Suicidal Adolescents

A recent review (Hawton et al. 1998) highlighted that children and adolescents who have engaged in deliberate self-harm have, almost exclusively, not been the direct focus of any systematic efforts to examine treatment outcome. The investigators described all randomized controlled trials that have evaluated the efficacy of treatments specifically targeting suicide attempters. Of the 20 studies reviewed, only one explicitly used an adolescent sample (Cotgrove et al. 1995). In that study, investigators compared suicide attempters assigned to standard care ($n=58$) with those who received standard care plus a token that ensured hospital readmission on demand ($n=47$). Rates of repeat suicide attempts were lower among subjects who received standard care plus the token, although this difference was not statistically significant.

More recently, Harrington and associates (Byford et al. 1999; Harrington et al. 1998a) conducted a randomized controlled trial of CBT that exclusively targeted child and adolescent suicide attempters ($N=162$) and their families. The study investigated both the efficacy and the effectiveness (i.e., clinical utility) of a very brief, home-based problem-solving intervention conducted by psychiatric social workers. Relative to routine care, the family-based intervention was equally cost-effective and showed better rates of compliance. However, results indicated no differences between patients assigned to these treatments on measures of suicidal ideation, hopelessness, and family functioning at 2- and 6-month follow-up. The family-based intervention did appear to result in a relative reduction of suicidal ideation for nondepressed patients.

Several innovative change strategies for adolescent suicide attempters have been described in the literature (see Brent and Lerner 1994; Freeman and Reinecke 1993; Kerfoot et al. 1995; Rotheram-Borus et al. 1994). Among these, time-limited, cognitive-behavioral interventions that incorporate some level of family involvement have been promoted most frequently, with most treatments focusing on development of adaptive coping strategies and problem-solving skills. More recently, researchers have begun to emphasize the relevance of broader social networks in suicide intervention (King et al. 2000).

In practical terms, such efforts are often considered secondary or tertiary interventions (Shaffer et al. 1988), insofar as treatment is designed to prevent recurrent episodes of suicidal behavior. The few empirically oriented treatment efficacy studies reported in the literature on adolescent suicide research have been limited to pilot investigations of treatment feasibility (i.e., open clinical trials). Other studies have used "mixed" clinical samples of attempters and ideators, nonrepresentative subgroups, or wholly analogue (i.e., nonclinical) populations (e.g., Gutstein and Rudd 1990).

Rudd et al. (1996) evaluated the efficacy of a time-limited group problem-solving therapy in a nonrepresentative (82% male) sample of 264 suicidal young adults (mean age=22 years), which included ideators (41.7% of the total) and single and repeat suicide attempters (40.5% and 17.8%, respectively). The intervention was provided on an outpatient basis, following a hospital day-treatment format (patients attended daily therapy sessions, each lasting up to 9 hours over a 2-week period), and was compared with treatment as usual. Immediately following treatment (1 month), both therapies were shown to be initially effective in 1) reducing levels of self-rated suicidal ideation, hopelessness, depressive symptomatology, and life stress; and 2) improving self-appraisal of general problem-solving abilities. At 6- and 12-month follow-up, patients showed similar rates of improvement across groups; no significant group differences were found on any of the same outcome measures.

In another study, Lerner and Clum (1990) assessed the relative efficacy of social problem-solving group therapy (based on D'Zurilla and Goldfried 1971) and supportive group therapy in a nonclinical (college student) sample of 18 suicide ideators, ranging in age from 18 to 24 years. The superiority of the problem-solving approach was indicated on widely used, self-report measures of depression, hopelessness, and loneliness at 3-month follow-up. However, no significant group differences were found on a measure of suicidal ideation and two different measures of problem-solving ability after 3 months.

Dialectical Behavior Therapy

Dialectical behavior therapy (DBT) is problem-oriented and complements direct change strategies (behavioral analysis, contingency management, cognitive restructuring) with acceptance strategies (validation, reciprocal communication). The treatment is broad-based, including multiple intervention modalities and components, designed to address the range of problem domains associated with suicidal behavior. Patients attend concurrent weekly individual and group skills training sessions for a 12-month period, while telephone consultation with the primary therapist is provided in crisis situations and to enhance skill generalization. Patients are trained to increase adaptive coping in four broad problem areas: identity confusion, impulsivity, emotion dysregulation, and interpersonal problems.

Linehan et al. (1991) showed the efficacy of a manual-based DBT intervention in a sample of 44 clinically referred repeat suicide attempters, all of whom met DSM-III (American Psychiatric Association 1980) diagnostic criteria for borderline personality disorder. Relative to control cases assigned to treatment as usual in the community, patients assigned to DBT engaged in significantly fewer and less severe parasuicidal behaviors at posttreatment (12 months). Attrition rates were significantly higher among control subjects (50%) than among DBT patients (17%). Subjects in the two groups showed comparable improvement in self-ratings of depression, hopelessness, suicidal ideation, and reasons for living.

More recently, Miller and associates (1997) adapted DBT for the treatment of suicidal adolescents with borderline features (DBT-A). The adaptation was characterized by several modifications: 1) participation of family members in skills training groups, 2) significantly shortened length of treatment (12 weeks), 3) focus on learning fewer adaptive skills, 4) an option to participate in a 12-week follow-up consultation group, and 5) use of simplified language in psychoeducational exercises to accommodate disadvantaged adolescents with below-average reading abilities. Rathus and Miller (in press) reported preliminary results of a nonrandomized controlled trial of DBT-A with 111 predominantly Hispanic adolescent outpatients ranging in age from 12 to 19 years. Participants were assigned to the adapted DBT treatment condition if they 1) had either attempted suicide in the preceding 16-week period or reported current suicidal ideation and 2) had at least three features of borderline personality disorder (i.e., DSM-IV-TR [American Psychiatric Association 2000] diagnostic criteria for a minimum of 1 year). Results indicated that the treatment was acceptable to adolescents and families and may have reduced the need for hospitalization during treatment. Controlled studies are needed to provide further support for the utility of this approach.

Summary of Interventions for Suicidal Youth

Innovative psychosocial interventions that specifically target suicidal thoughts and self-harm behaviors in clinically referred adolescents are especially desirable considering the potential for deliberate overdose that pharmacological interventions carry. Despite the public health significance of youth suicide, no effective psychotherapeutic treatments are currently available for high-risk adolescents. At least one study has found that DBT may be effective for suicidal adults (Linehan et al. 1991). Observed reductions in the frequency of suicide attempts in this study may be attributable to higher baseline attempt rates characteristic of patients with borderline personality disorder. Thus, Linehan et al.'s findings may not generalize to suicidal patients who do not meet criteria for borderline personality disorder.

Nevertheless, downward extensions of DBT may be of value. In fact, preliminary data suggest that DBT-A, an abbreviated adaptation of Linehan et al.'s protocol, may be effective in reducing the frequency of hospitalization among suicidal adolescents with borderline traits. Future research should focus on evaluating the efficacy of DBT-A in controlled clinical trials that include adolescents with more heterogeneous diagnostic profiles. Interventionists must develop a more sophisticated understanding of the challenges to the conduct of suicide intervention research and, despite them, should be encouraged to initiate clinical psychotherapy trials that target suicidal adolescents.

Implications for Future Research on Psychotherapy for Depressed and Suicidal Youth

Although research in child and adolescent depression still lags behind that of adult depression, significant strides are being made. The state of treatment research for suicidal youth is further behind still. For depression, the recovery, relapse, and recurrence rates cited suggest that there is room for the development of other effective treatments and for enhancing the effectiveness of the extant treatments. Specific areas in need of further investigation include 1) comparison studies of multiple active treatments, 2) comparison of psychotherapy with medication, 3) studies of combination treatment strategies, and 4) studies of sequential or modular treatments. Populations in need of study include 1) clinically referred prepubertal children meeting full criteria for a depression diagnosis and 2) depressed children and adolescents with varying comorbid disorders other than anxiety disorders. Studies also need to include more broad-based outcomes so that efficacy is confirmed not only for reduction of depressive symptoms but also for functioning in different domains of the adolescents' lives such as at school, with peers, and with family. Finally, clinical trials must not be limited to university clinic settings and must be conducted in community settings in which treatment is more commonly delivered such as school clinics and primary care settings. For suicidal youth, the field is open and waiting for investigators to rise to the challenge of studying the efficacy of existing psychosocial treatments such as adapted DBT and for the development of new treatment approaches for this significant public health problem.

References

American Academy of Child and Adolescent Psychiatry: Practice parameters for the assessment and treatment of children and adolescents with depressive disorders. J Am Acad Child Adolesc Psychiatry 37:10 (suppl):63S–83S, 1998

American Academy of Child and Adolescent Psychiatry: Practice parameters for the assessment and treatment of children and adolescents with suicidal behavior. J Am Acad Child Adolesc Psychiatry 40 (suppl):24–51, 2001

American Psychiatric Association: Diagnostic and Statistical Manual of Mental Disorders, 3rd Edition. Washington, DC, American Psychiatric Association, 1980

American Psychiatric Association: Diagnostic and Statistical Manual of Mental Disorders, 3rd Edition, Revised. Washington, DC, American Psychiatric Association, 1987

American Psychiatric Association: Diagnostic and Statistical Manual of Mental Disorders, 4th Edition, Text Revision. Washington, DC, American Psychiatric Association, 2000

Andrews JA, Lewinsohn PM: Suicidal attempts among older adolescents: prevalence and co-occurrence with psychiatric disorders. J Am Acad Child Adolesc Psychiatry 31:655–662, 1992

Aseltine R, Gore S, Colten M: Depression and the social developmental context of adolescence. J Pers Soc Psychol 67:252–263, 1994

Beck AT, Rush AJ, Shaw BF, et al: Cognitive Therapy of Depression. New York, Guilford, 1979

Birmaher B, Brent DA, Kolko D, et al: Clinical outcome after short-term psychotherapy for adolescents with major depressive disorder. Arch Gen Psychiatry 57:29–36, 2000

Brent DA, Lerner MS: Cognitive therapy with affectively ill, suicidal adolescents, in Cognitive Therapy for Depressed Adolescents. Edited by Wilkes TCR, Belsher G, Rush AJ, et al. New York, Guilford, 1994, pp 298–320

Brent DA, Perper JA, Moritz G, et al: Psychiatric risk factors for adolescent suicide: a case-control study. J Am Acad Child Adolesc Psychiatry 32:521–529, 1993

Brent DA, Holder D, Kolko D, et al: A clinical psychotherapy trial for adolescent depression comparing cognitive, family and supportive treatments. Arch Gen Psychiatry 54:877–885, 1997

Brent DA, Kolko D, Birmaher B, et al: Predictors of treatment efficacy in a clinical trial of three psychosocial treatments for adolescent depression. J Am Acad Child Adolesc Psychiatry 37:906–914, 1998

Butler L, Miezitis S, Friedman R, et al: The effect of two school-based intervention programs on depressive symptoms in preadolescents. American Educational Research Journal 17:111–119, 1980

Byford S, Harrington R, Torgerson D, et al: Cost-effectiveness analysis of a home-based social work intervention for children and adolescents who have deliberately poisoned themselves: results of a randomised controlled trial. Br J Psychiatry 174:56–62, 1999

Centers for Disease Control and Prevention: Youth Risk Behavior Surveillance—United States, 1999. MMWR Morb Mortal Wkly Rep 49:1–95, 2000

Clarke G, Hops H, Lewinsohn PM, et al: Cognitive-behavioral group treatment of adolescent depression: prediction of outcome. Behavior Therapy 23:341–354, 1992

Clarke GN, Hawkins W, Murphy M, et al: School-based primary prevention of depressive symptomatology in adolescents: findings from two studies. Journal of Adolescent Research 8:183–321, 1993

Clarke GN, Hawkins W, Murphy M, et al: Targeted prevention of unipolar depressive disorder in an at-risk sample of high school adolescents: a randomized trial of a group cognitive intervention. J Am Acad Child Adolesc Psychiatry 34:312–321, 1995

Clarke GN, Lewinsohn PM, Rohde P, et al: Cognitive-behavioral group treatment of adolescent depression: efficacy of acute group treatment and booster sessions. J Am Acad Child Adolesc Psychiatry 38:272–279, 1999

Cotgrove A, Zirinsky L, Black D, et al: Secondary prevention of attempted suicide in adolescence. J Adolesc 18:569–577, 1995

Diamond G, Siqueland L: Family therapy for the treatment of depressed adolescents. Family Therapy 32:77–90, 1995

DiMascio A, Klerman GL, Weissman MM, et al: A control group for psychotherapy research in acute depression: one solution to ethical and methodological issues. J Psychiatr Res 15:189–197, 1979

D'Zurilla TJ, Goldfried MR: Problem solving and behavior modification. J Abnorm Psychol 78:107–126, 1971

Elkin I, Shea MT, Watkins JT, et al: National Institute of Mental Health Treatment of Depression Collaborative Research Program: general effectiveness of treatments. Arch Gen Psychiatry 45:971–983, 1989

Emery G, Bedrosian R, Garber J: Cognitive therapy with depressed children and adolescents, in Affective Disorders in Childhood and Adolescence—An Update. Edited by Cantwell DP, Carlson GA. New York, Spectrum Publications, 1983, pp 445–471

Ferro T, Verdeli H, Pierre F, et al: Screening for depression in mothers bringing their offspring for evaluation or treatment of depression. Am J Psychiatry 157:375–379, 2000

Fine S, Forth A, Gilbert M, et al: Group therapy for adolescent depressive disorder: a comparison of social skills and therapeutic support. J Am Acad Child Adolesc Psychiatry 30:79–85, 1991

Freeman A, Reinecke MA: Cognitive Therapy of Suicidal Behavior: A Manual for Treatment. New York, Springer, 1993

Fristad MA, Gavazzi SM, Soldano KW: Multi-family psychoeducation groups for childhood mood disorders. Contemporary Family Therapy 20:385–402, 1998

Garber J, Weiss B, Shanley N: Cognitions, depressive symptoms, and development in adolescents. J Abnorm Psychol 102:47–57, 1993

Gilham JE, Reivich KJ, Jaycox LH, et al: Prevention of depressive symptoms in schoolchildren: a two year follow-up. Psychological Science 6:343–351, 1995

Gould MS, Fisher P, Parides M, et al: Psychosocial risk factors of child and adolescent completed suicide. Arch Gen Psychiatry 53:1155–1162, 1996

Gould MS, King R, Greenwald S, et al: Psychopathology associated with suicidal ideation and attempts among children and adolescents. J Am Acad Child Adolesc Psychiatry 37:915–923, 1998

Greenhill LL, Waslick B: Management of suicidal behavior in children and adolescents. Psychiatr Clin North Am 20:641–666, 1997

Gutheil TG: Liability issues and liability prevention in suicide, in The Harvard Medical School Guide to Suicidal Assessment and Interventions. Edited by Jacobs DG. San Francisco, CA, Jossey-Bass, 1999, pp 561–578

Gutstein SE, Rudd MD: An outpatient treatment alternative for suicidal youth. J Adolesc 13:265–277, 1990

Hammen C: The emergence of an interpersonal approach to depression, in The Interactional Nature of Depression: Advances in Interpersonal Approaches. Edited by Joiner T, Coyne J. Washington, DC, American Psychological Association, 1999, pp 22–36

Harrington R, Kerfoot M, Dyer E, et al: Randomized trial of a home-based family intervention for children who have deliberately poisoned themselves. J Am Acad Child Adolesc Psychiatry 37:512–518, 1998a

Harrington R, Whittaker J, Shoebridge P: Psychological treatment of depression in children and adolescents: a review of treatment research. Br J Psychiatry 173:291–298, 1998b

Hawton K, Arensman E, Townsend E, et al: Deliberate self harm: systematic review of efficacy of psychosocial and pharmacological treatments in preventing repetition. BMJ 317:441–447, 1998

Hoagwood K, Hibbs E, Brent D, et al: Introduction to the special section: efficacy and effectiveness in studies of child and adolescent psychotherapy. J Consult Clin Psychol 63:683–687, 1995

Jaycox LH, Reivich KJ, Gilham J, et al: Preventing depressive symptoms in school children. Behav Res Ther 32:801–816, 1994

Jayson D, Wood A, Kroll L, et al: Which depressed patients respond to cognitive-behavioral treatment? J Am Acad Child Adolesc Psychiatry 37:35–39, 1998

Joiner T, Coyne J, Blalock J: On the interpersonal nature of depression: overview and synthesis, in The Interactional Nature of Depression: Advances in Interpersonal Approaches. Edited by Joiner T, Coyne J. Washington, DC, American Psychological Association, 1999, pp 3–20

Kahn JS, Kehle TJ, Jenson WR, et al: Comparison of cognitive-behavioral relaxation training, and self-modeling interventions for depression among middle school students. School Psychology Review 27:146–155, 1990

Kaslow NJ, Thompson MP: Applying the criteria for empirically supported treatments to studies of psychosocial interventions for child and adolescent depression. J Clin Child Psychol 27:146–155, 1998

Kerfoot M, Harrington R, Dyer E: Brief home-based intervention with young suicide attempters and their families. J Adolesc 18:557–568, 1995

King CA, Hovey JD, Brand E, et al: Suicidal adolescents after hospitalization: parent and family impacts on treatment follow-through. J Am Acad Child Adolesc Psychiatry 36:85–93, 1997

King C, Preuss L, Kramer A, et al: Connect five: a social network intervention for suicidal youth. Poster presented at the 47th annual meeting of the American Academy of Child and Adolescent Psychiatry, New York, October 2000

Klerman G, Weissman MM, Rounsaville B, et al: Interpersonal Psychotherapy of Depression. New York, Basic Books, 1984

Kovacs M: The Children's Depression Inventory. Psychopharmacol Bull 21:995–998, 1985

Kovacs M: Depressive disorders in childhood: an impressionistic landscape. J Child Psychol Psychiatry 38:287–298, 1997

Kroll L, Harrington R, Jayson D, et al: Pilot study of continuation cognitive-behavioral therapy for major depression in adolescent psychiatric patients. J Am Acad Child Adolesc Psychiatry 35:1156–1161, 1996

Lerner MS, Clum GA: Treatment of suicide ideators: a problem-solving approach. Behavior Therapy 21:403–411, 1990

Lewinsohn PM, Clarke GN: Psychosocial treatments for adolescent depression. Clin Psychol Rev 19:329–342, 1999

Lewinsohn PM, Weinstein M, Shaw D: Depression: a clinical-research approach, in Advances in Behavior Therapy. Edited by Rubin R, Frank C. New York, Academic Press, 1969, pp 231–240

Lewinsohn PM, Antonuccio DO, Steinmetz J, et al: The Coping With Depression Course: A Psychoeducational Intervention for Unipolar Depression. Eugene, OR, Castalia Press, 1984

Lewinsohn PM, Clarke GN, Hops H, et al: Cognitive-behavioral treatment for depressed adolescents. Behavior Therapy 21:385–401, 1990

Lewinsohn PM, Clarke GN, Rohde P, et al: A course in coping: a cognitive-behavioral approach to the treatment of adolescent depression, in Psychosocial Treatments for Child and Adolescent Disorders: Empirically Based Strategies for Clinical Practice. Edited by Hibbs ED, Jensen PS. Washington, DC, American Psychiatric Press, 1996, pp 109–135

Liddle BJ, Spence SH: Cognitive-behavioral therapy with depressed primary school children: a cautionary note. Behavioral Psychotherapy 18:85–102, 1990

Linehan MM, Armstrong HE, Suarez A, et al: Cognitive-behavioral treatment of chronically parasuicidal borderline patients. Arch Gen Psychiatry 48:1060–1064, 1991

Miller AL, Rathus JH, Linehan MM, et al: Dialectical behavior therapy adapted for suicidal adolescents. Journal of Practical Psychiatry and Behavioral Health 3:78–86, 1997

Mueller C, Orvaschel H: The failure of "adult" interventions with adolescent depression: what does it mean for theory, research and practice? J Affect Disord 44:203–215, 1997

Mufson L, Fairbanks J: Interpersonal psychotherapy for depressed adolescents: a one year naturalistic follow-up study. J Am Acad Child Adolesc Psychiatry 35:1145–1155, 1996

Mufson L, Moreau D, Weissman MM, et al: Interpersonal Psychotherapy for Depressed Adolescents. New York, Guilford, 1993

Mufson L, Moreau D, Weissman MM, et al: The modification of interpersonal psychotherapy with depressed adolescents IPT-A: Phase I and Phase II studies. J Am Acad Child Adolesc Psychiatry 33:695–705, 1994

Mufson L, Weissman MM, Moreau D, et al: Efficacy of interpersonal psychotherapy for depressed adolescents. Arch Gen Psychiatry 56:573–579, 1999

Pearson JL, Stanley B, King C, et al: Issues to consider in intervention research with persons at high risk for suicidality. National Institute of Mental Health Web site. Available at: http://www.nimh.nih.gov/research/highrisksuicide.cfm. Accessed 2001.

Piacentini J, Rotheram-Borus MJ, Gillis JR, et al: Demographic predictors of treatment attendance among adolescent suicide attempters. J Consult Clin Psychol 63:469–473, 1995

Poznanski EO, Mokros HB: Children's Depression Rating Scale, Revised (CDRS-R): Manual. Los Angeles, CA, Western Psychological Services, 1996

Puig-Antich J, Lukens E, Davies M, et al: Psychosocial functioning in prepubertal major depressive disorders, I: interpersonal relationships during the depressive episode. Arch Gen Psychiatry 42:500–507, 1985

Puig-Antich J, Kaufman J, Ryan ND, et al: The psychosocial functioning and family environment of depressed adolescents. J Am Acad Child Adolesc Psychiatry 32:244–253, 1993

Rathus JH, Miller AL: Dialectical behavior therapy adapted for suicidal adolescents: a pilot study. Suicide Life Threat Behav (in press)

Reinecke MA, Ryan NE, DuBois DL: Cognitive-behavioral therapy of depression and depressive symptoms during adolescence: a review and meta-analysis. J Am Acad Child Adolesc Psychiatry 37:26–34, 1998

Reynolds WM, Coates KI: A comparison of cognitive-behavioral therapy and relaxation training for the treatment of depression in adolescents. J Consult Clin Psychol 54:653–660, 1986

Rossello J, Bernal G: The efficacy of cognitive-behavioral and interpersonal treatments for depression in Puerto Rican adolescents. J Consult Clin Psychol 67:734–745, 1999

Rotheram-Borus MJ, Piacentini J, Miller S, et al: Brief cognitive-behavioral treatment for adolescent suicide attempters and their families. J Am Acad Child Adolesc Psychiatry 33:508–517, 1994

Rotheram-Borus MJ, Piacentini J, Van Rossem R, et al: Enhancing treatment adherence with a specialized emergency room program for adolescent suicide attempters. J Am Acad Child Adolesc Psychiatry 35:654–663, 1996a

Rotheram-Borus MJ, Walker JU, Ferns W: Suicidal behavior among middle-class adolescents who seek crisis services. J Clin Psychol 52:137–143, 1996b

Rotheram-Borus MJ, Piacentini J, Van Rossem R, et al: Treatment adherence among Latina female adolescent suicide attempters. Suicide Life Threat Behav 29:319–331, 1999

Rudd MD, Rajab MH, Orman DT, et al: Effectiveness of an outpatient intervention targeting suicidal young adults: preliminary results. J Consult Clin Psychol 64:179–190, 1996

Rudd MD, Joiner T, Rajab MH: Treating Suicidal Behavior: An Effective, Time-limited Approach. New York, Guilford, 2000

Shaffer D, Garland A, Gould M, et al: Preventing teenage suicide: a critical review. J Am Acad Child Adolesc Psychiatry 27:675–687, 1988

Shaffer D, Gould MS, Fisher P, et al: Psychiatric diagnosis in child and adolescent suicide. Arch Gen Psychiatry 53:339–348, 1996

Spirito A, Brown L, Overholser J, et al: Attempted suicide in adolescence: a review and critique of the literature. Clin Psychol Rev 9:335–363, 1989

Spirito A, Plummer B, Gispert M, et al: Adolescent suicide attempts: outcomes at follow-up. Am J Orthopsychiatry 62:464–468, 1992

Stader S, Hokanson J: Psychological antecedents of depressive symptoms: an evaluation using daily experiences methodology. J Abnorm Psychol 107:17–26, 1998

Stark KD, Reynolds WM, Kaslow NJ: A comparison of the relative efficacy of self-control therapy and a behavioral problem-solving therapy for depression in children. J Abnorm Child Psychol 15:91–113, 1987

Stark KD, Rouse LW, Livingston R: Treatment of depression during childhood and adolescence: cognitive and behavioral procedures for the individual and family, in Child and Adolescent Therapy: Cognitive-Behavioral Procedures. Edited by Kendall PC. New York, Guilford, 1991, pp 165–206

Task Force on Promotion and Dissemination of Psychological Procedures: Training in and dissemination of empirically validated psychological treatments: report and recommendations. The Clinical Psychologist 8:3–24, 1996

Trautman PD, Stewart N, Morishima A: Are adolescent suicide attempters noncompliant with outpatient care? J Am Acad Child Adolesc Psychiatry 32:89–94, 1993

Vostanis P, Feehan C, Grattan E, et al: A randomized controlled outpatient trial of cognitive-behavioral treatment for children and adolescents with depression: 9 month follow-up. J Affect Disord 40:105–116, 1996a

Vostanis P, Feehan C, Grattan E, et al: Treatment for children and adolescents with depression: lessons from a controlled trial. Clin Child Psychol Psychiatry 1:199–212, 1996b

Weissman MM, Prusoff BA, DiMascio A, et al: The efficacy of drug and psychotherapy in the treatment of acute depressive episodes. Am J Psychiatry 136:555–558, 1979

Weisz JR, Thurber CA, Sweeney L, et al: Brief treatment of mild-to-moderate child depression using primary and secondary control enhancement training. J Consult Clin Psychol 65:703–707, 1997

Wood A, Harrington R, Moore A: Controlled trial of a brief cognitive-behavioral intervention in adolescent patients with depressive disorders. J Child Psychol Psychiatry 37:737–746, 1996

Chapter 3

Pharmacotherapy for Depression in Children and Adolescents

Boris Birmaher, M.D.
David Brent, M.D.

Major depressive disorder (MDD) is a familial recurrent illness associated with increased risk for suicidal behavior and suicide attempts, other psychiatric disorders (e.g., substance abuse), poor psychosocial and academic outcome, and depression and psychological difficulties during adulthood (Birmaher et al. 1996a; Pine et al. 1998; Rao et al. 1999; Weissman et al. 1999). The prevalence of MDD in children and adolescents is approximately 2% and 6%, respectively (Birmaher et al. 1996a). Thus, early identification and prompt treatment of this disorder at its early stages is critical.

The main goal of the pharmacological treatment is to achieve remission and prevent relapses and depressive recurrences (for definitions, see Table 3–1).

In this chapter, we review the current pharmacological management for the acute, continuation, and maintenance treatment phases of MDD in children and adolescents (American Academy of Child and Adolescent Psychiatry 1998; American Psychiatric Association 2000). In addition, we review the pharmacological management of treatment-resistant MDD.

Supported in part by National Institute of Mental Health grants MH55123, MH70008, and MH 61835.

Table 3–1. Definitions of treatment response

Absence of MDD	≤1 symptom of MDD
Subsyndromal depression	2–3 symptoms of MDD
Response	No MDD or a significant reduction in the MDD symptoms for at least 2 weeks (e.g., a 50% reduction in symptomatology from baseline, a Children's Depression Rating Scale, Revised, score ≤ 28, Beck Depression Inventory score ≤ 9)
Remission	A period of at least 2 weeks and <2 months with absence of MDD
Recovery	Absence of MDD for ≥2 months
Relapse	An episode of depression during the period of remission
Recurrence	The emergence of symptoms of MDD during the period of recovery (a new episode)

Note.   MDD = major depressive disorder.

The *acute phase* for a youngster with the first episode of depression usually lasts 6–12 weeks. The main goals during this phase are to achieve response and remission of the depressive symptoms. The *continuation phase* usually lasts 6–12 months, during which remission is consolidated to prevent relapses. The *maintenance phase* lasts 1 or more years, and its main goal is the prevention of depression recurrences. Most of the studies in children and adolescents have evaluated the response to antidepressants during the acute phase, with no controlled trials in continuation or maintenance phases. Therefore, recommendations regarding the continuation and maintenance treatments are extrapolated from the adult literature, but caution is warranted because youths may respond differently to continuation and maintenance interventions thus far only tested in adults with MDD (Birmaher et al. 1996b).

Acute Phase Treatment

The published pharmacological studies of acute phase treatment in children and adolescents have focused on the effects of the tricyclic antidepressants (TCAs) and, more recently, the selective serotonin reuptake inhibitors (SSRIs). Other antidepressants, including the heterocyclics (e.g., amoxapine, maprotiline), bupropion, venlafaxine, mirtazapine, nefazodone, and the monoamine oxidase inhibitors (MAOIs), have been found to be efficacious for the treatment of depressed adults (American Psychiatric Association 2000), but they have not been well studied for the treatment of MDD in children and adolescents. However, in some cases, controlled studies are under way. Therefore, we describe mainly the use of SSRIs and TCAs for youths with MDD.

Selective Serotonin Reuptake Inhibitors

SSRIs have become the first-line pharmacological treatment of depression across ages because of their reported efficacy (American Psychiatric Association 2000; Emslie et al. 1997; Keller et al. 2001) and their relatively benign side-effect profile. One of the most important aspects of this favorable side-effect profile is a much lower risk of fatality in overdose compared with TCAs (Kapur et al. 1992).

The SSRIs also have been shown to be efficacious and well tolerated in the treatment of pediatric anxiety and obsessive-compulsive disorders (March et al. 1998; Research Units of Pediatric Psychopharmacology Anxiety Group 2001).

The SSRIs selectively block the presynaptic neuronal reuptake of serotonin with mild or no affinity for the adrenergic, cholinergic, or histaminergic receptors (Leonard et al. 1997; Preskorn 1999). In adults, all SSRIs appear to be equally efficacious for the treatment of major depression, and overall they present similar side effects. However, they differ with respect to elimination half-lives, drug interactions, and the antidepressant activity of their metabolites (Axelson et al. 2000a, 2000b; Findling et al. 1999; Preskorn 1999).

Open studies with SSRIs for depressed children and adolescents have reported a 70%–90% response rate (e.g., Ambrosini et al. 1999). A double-blind, placebo-controlled study in a very small sample of adolescents with MDD did not find significant differences between placebo and fluoxetine (Simeon et al. 1990).

However, a large 8-week double-blind study of the treatment of MDD in children and adolescents showed that patients receiving 8 weeks of fluoxetine (20 mg/day) were more likely to show improvement than were those receiving placebo (58% vs. 32% on the Clinical Global Impression Improvement subscale [CGI-S]) (Emslie et al. 1997). A second multisite study that also used fluoxetine (20 mg/day) for 9 weeks replicated the above results, with fluoxetine being superior to placebo (40% vs. 20%, $P=0.01$). A Children's Depression Rating Scale, Revised (CDRS-R) score of 28 or less and a CGI-I score improvement of 2 or less were used as the definitions of response (Emslie et al. 2000). In both studies, no age and sex effects were seen, and patients tolerated the fluoxetine well. Despite the significant response to fluoxetine, many patients had only partial improvement, and only about one-third experienced complete symptomatic relief (Emslie et al. 1997). This low rate of complete response may be a result of inadequate duration of treatment. In fact, in naturalistic follow-up, Emslie et al. (1998) did find that the proportion who responded increased as the treatment continued. In addition, the dosage of fluoxetine in this study may not have been adequate for all subjects. In adults, some evidence indicates that a higher dosage of fluoxetine may improve symptomatic response (Fava et al. 1995). For more severe or chronic depression, the optimal treatment might require a combination of pharmacological and psychosocial treatments, as has been suggested in studies of chronic depression in adults (Keller et al. 2000).

A recent multicenter study compared the effects of paroxetine (mean dose at study end=28 ± 8.5 mg/day), imipramine (mean dose=205 ± 64 mg/day), and placebo for the treatment of MDD in a large sample of outpatient adolescents ($N=275$) over 12 weeks (Keller et al. 2001). Adolescents taking paroxetine showed significantly better response than did those taking placebo (CGI-I score ≤2: 65.6% vs. 48.3%, $P=0.02$). No differences were found between the youths taking imipramine and placebo, and importantly, this trial was the first placebo-controlled study with TCAs that was adequately powered to accept the null hypothesis that TCAs were no different from placebo. Approximately 31.5% of the patients taking imipramine were removed from the study for side effects in comparison with only 9.7% of those taking paroxetine.

In the above-noted studies, nonresponse was associated with comorbid dysthymia, attention-deficit/hyperactivity disorder (ADHD), or anxiety; severity of depression; and family conflict (Birmaher et al. 2000a; Emslie et al. 1998).

In adults and in youths, the time course of improvement with the SSRIs appears to be similar (American Psychiatric Association 2000; Emslie et al. 1998). Therefore, after 4–6 weeks, if a patient has only a partial response, the dose may be increased.

Side Effects

Overall, all SSRIs have similar side-effect profiles, and patients tend to develop tolerance to some of these side effects over time. Although the SSRIs do not show a clear dose-response relationship, most of the side effects *are* dose dependent (Preskorn 1999). The most frequent side effects are gastrointestinal symptoms (e.g., nausea, diarrhea), decreased appetite, decreased or (more controversial) increased weight, headaches, restlessness, jitteriness, tremor, insomnia or hypersomnia, diaphoresis, vivid dreams, and sexual dysfunction (painful or delayed ejaculation, anorgasmia). Similar to other antidepressants, SSRIs may trigger an episode of hypomania or mania in vulnerable patients, but clinicians should be able to differentiate these symptoms from akathisia, jitteriness, and the so-called behavioral activation (agitation and disinhibition) (Wilens et al. 1998). Allergic reactions have been reported, but, as with any other medications, these need to be differentiated from allergies to the dyes contained in the medications. The SSRIs have been implicated in inducing extrapyramidal symptoms and hyponatremia, and they have been associated with ecchymoses (American Psychiatric Association 2000; Lake et al. 2000; Leonard et al. 1997).

Discontinuation

Especially with SSRIs with shorter half-lives (e.g., paroxetine, fluvoxamine), sudden or rapid cessation may induce withdrawal symptoms that can mimic a relapse or recurrence of a depressive episode (e.g., tiredness, irritability). Furthermore, one clinical impression is that rapid discontinuation of antidepressants may induce relapses or recurrences of depression. Therefore, if these medications need to be discontinued, they should be tapered gradually, over a period of at least 2 weeks.

Pharmacokinetic Studies

In children and adolescents, the steady-state half-lives of antidepressants such as paroxetine, sertraline, and citalopram at common therapeutic doses are between 14 and 16 hours, which is significantly shorter than has been reported in adults (Axelson et al. 2000a, 2000b; Findling et al. 1999). This suggests that, at least at lower doses, these medications may need to be prescribed twice a day. Otherwise, children and adolescents can experience withdrawal side effects during the evening, and these symptoms can be confused with lack of response or medication side effects. One study suggested that sertraline, at doses of 200 mg/day, can be prescribed once a day (Alderman et al. 1998), but further studies are necessary. Pharmacokinetic studies with the other antidepressants are necessary because youths appear to metabolize these medications faster than adults do, and therefore dose frequency guidelines for adults may need to be modified for pediatric patients.

Pharmacogenetic Studies

No pharmacogenetic studies of the prediction of SSRI response in children and adolescents have been done, but there are some promising results in adults. The short form of the serotonin transporter gene has been associated with nonresponse, or a less vigorous response, to SSRIs in mid- and late-life depressive patients (e.g., Pollock et al. 2000). In addition, a recent report found an association with this polymorphism and switch to mania during treatment of depression (Mundo et al. 2001).

Interactions With Other Medications

All SSRIs and their metabolites (Leonard et al. 1997; Preskorn 1999) are metabolized in different degrees by the hepatic cytochrome P450 enzymes. Of the five major cytochrome P450 enzymes mediating the oxidative drug metabolism, CYP3A3/4 and

CYP2D6 are responsible for approximately 50% and 30% of known oxidative drug metabolism, respectively (Preskorn 1999). Except for citalopram and sertraline, the currently available SSRIs are mainly metabolized by the CYP3A3/4 and CYP2D6 enzymes. Substantial inhibition of these isoenzymes converts a normal metabolizer into a slow metabolizer with regard to this specific pathway. Therefore, it is important to be aware of the possibility that toxicity could result if other medications are prescribed that are also metabolized by the cytochrome P450 system, such as the TCAs, neuroleptics, atypical antipsychotics, antiarrhythmics, antihypertensives, theophylline, terfenadine, benzodiazepines, carbamazepine, and warfarin (Preskorn 1999).

The SSRIs also have a high degree of protein binding, which may lead to increased therapeutic or toxic effects of other protein-bound medications.

SSRIs should be stopped before initiating treatment with MAOIs to avoid precipitating a serotonin syndrome. After discontinuation of the SSRI, an MAOI should not be started for at least 2 weeks for all SSRIs except fluoxetine, which, because of its long half-life, requires 5 weeks before MAOI treatment can be initiated. Also, the SSRIs should not be administered for at least 2 weeks after stopping an MAOI.

Tricyclic Antidepressants

Studies in depressed adults involving thousands of subjects have shown approximately a 50%–70% response to TCAs, with drug-placebo differences ranging from 20% to 40% (American Psychiatric Association 2000). In contrast, only 13 double-blind psychopharmacological trials, which included approximately 330 depressed children and adolescents, comparing TCAs (nortriptyline, imipramine, desipramine, amitriptyline) with placebo have been reported. These studies showed similar responses to both the TCAs and placebo (for a review, see Birmaher et al. 1996b). The above-noted studies need to be considered as preliminary because of methodological limitations—in particular, small sample sizes; short-duration trials; and inclusion of patients with mild depressions, lower levels of neurovegetative symptoms, and comorbid disorders that may have higher response to placebo (Birmaher et al. 1996b). However, a recent study comparing imipramine, paroxetine, and placebo (Keller et al. 2001) in a sample of adolescents with MDD sufficiently large to accept the null hypothesis reported no significant differences between imipramine and placebo, indicating that the TCAs are not the first-line medication for the treatment of MDD in youths. However, it is important to emphasize that some individual patients may selectively respond to TCAs and not the newer antidepressants. Specifically, the TCAs may be indicated for the augmentation of the SSRIs (American Psychiatric Association 2000) and for the treatment of comorbid MDD and ADHD (Hughes et al. 1999). A recent report suggested that imipramine may be helpful, in combination with cognitive-behavioral therapy, for treatment of school-refusing adolescents with a combination of MDD and anxiety disorders (Bernstein et al. 2000).

Other Antidepressants

Other antidepressants, including bupropion, venlafaxine, nefazodone, and mirtazapine, have been found efficacious for the treatment of depression in adults, but only a few open studies of treatment in children and adolescents have been published (e.g., Daviss et al. 2001). Randomized controlled trials with some of these compounds are under way.

Bupropion may be useful in treating youths with MDD and ADHD (Daviss et al. 2001). Because of the sedative effects of mirtazapine and trazodone, these medications have been used as adjunctive treatment for patients with severe insomnia.

Treatment of Subtypes of Major Depressive Disorder

Psychotic Depression

Overall, only 20%–40% of the adults with psychotic MDD respond to antidepressant monotherapy, and the range of placebo response is from very low to null (American Psychiatric Association 2000). Although monotherapy with antidepressants may be effective, recovery appears to be both more robust and more rapid when antidepressants are combined with an antipsychotic. However, the long-term use of the typical neuroleptics has not been evaluated and carries the risk for tardive dyskinesia. Therefore, the antipsychotic should be tapered after remission of the depression. The newer antipsychotic medications (e.g., risperidone, olanzapine) may prove to be useful alternatives to the typical neuroleptics and deserve further investigation, especially because they have a secondary effect as a serotonin type 2 receptor agonist. Electroconvulsive therapy (ECT) is particularly effective for this subtype of depression in adults, but it has not been well studied in depressed youths (American Psychiatric Association 2000; Rey and Walter 1997).

Atypical Depression

Adult patients with atypical depression respond significantly better to the MAOIs and SSRIs than to the TCAs (American Psychiatric Association 2000). However, this has not been studied in younger patients.

Seasonal Affective Disorder

Studies in adults and a few studies in children and adolescents have suggested that bright-light therapy is efficacious for the treatment of seasonal affective disorder (see review by Swedo et al. 1997). The most widely used protocol consists of using the light box with 10,000 lux at 1-foot distance from the face of the patient for 30–45 minutes. Treatment can be extended to 1 hour in cases of partial response. Studies of light visors and other head-mounted devices have been controversial. Also, it is unclear at which time of the day light exposure is more efficacious, but some patients may respond better during the morning hours. However, morning treatment sessions may be difficult during the school calendar and for adolescents who refuse to wake up early. Bright-light therapy has been associated with some side effects such as headaches and "eye strain." Some authors have recommended an ophthalmological evaluation before initiating light therapy, but this practice has been frequently questioned unless patients have previous eye illnesses. Treatment with light may induce episodes of hypomania or mania in vulnerable patients.

Bipolar Depression

Most of the youths consulting for treatment of depression are experiencing their first depressive episode (Birmaher et al. 1996b). Because the symptoms of unipolar and bipolar depression are similar, it is difficult to decide whether a patient needs only an antidepressant or concomitant use of mood stabilizers. Some symptoms and signs such as psychosis, psychomotor retardation, and family history of bipolar disorder may warn the clinician about the risk of the child developing a manic episode (e.g., Geller et al. 1993; Strober and Carlson 1982).

No studies have been done in youths with bipolar depression, and few controlled pharmacological studies have been done in adults (Compton and Nemeroff 2000). Given the possibility that antidepressants may induce mania or rapid cycling, it has been recommended to start first with a mood stabilizer (lithium carbonate, valproate, carbamazepine) (American Psychiatric Association 1994) and then, if necessary, add an antidepressant. However, some adult studies have reported that antidepressant monotherapy may be appropriate (Amsterdam and Garcia-España 2000; Amsterdam et al. 1998), particularly for bipolar II patients with sporadic periods of hypomania, who may respond to an SSRI or bupropion, without mood stabilizers. However, although bipolar II disorder appears to be relatively stable in adults and unlikely to progress to full-blown mania, this may not be the case in adolescents, whose bipolar course may very well begin with brief hypomanic episodes (Lewinsohn et al. 2000). Furthermore, clinicians should be aware that antidepressants might induce rapid cycling in some bipolar patients.

In adults, mood stabilizers reduce the risk of cycling and have modest antidepressant effects (30%–50%) (American Psychiatric Association 1994). For patients with bipolar depression who do not respond to mood stabilizers alone, an antidepressant should be added to the treatment. Adult bipolar depressed patients may be less likely to respond to TCAs than are patients with unipolar depression (Himmelhoch et al. 1991). They may show a more favorable response to bupropion, SSRIs, and MAOIs. Furthermore, some studies, but not all, have suggested that, in comparison with other antidepressants, bupropion and the MAOIs are less likely to produce mania and rapid cycling (American Psychiatric Association 1994; Compton and Nemeroff 2000).

It is not clear how long a patient with bipolar depression should be treated with these medications, and studies are warranted. Recurrence rates of bipolar depression of approximately 60% have been observed in adult patients taking adequate doses of lithium, alone or together with imipramine (American Psychiatric Association 1994). TCAs are not indicated for bipolar depression in light of their lack of efficacy for youth unipolar depression and adult bipolar depression, as well as their likelihood of inducing rapid cycling in adults with bipolar disorder (American Psychiatric Association 1994, 2000; Birmaher et al. 1996b; Keller et al., in press). It remains to be seen whether the combination of mood stabilizers and other antidepressants such as bupropion and SSRIs yields more complete prophylaxis for youths with bipolar disorder.

Treatment of Comorbid Conditions and Suicidality

Comorbid disorders may influence the onset, maintenance, and recurrence of depression (Birmaher et al. 1996a, 1996b). Therefore, in addition to the treatment of depressive symptoms, it is of prime importance to treat the comorbid conditions that frequently accompany the depressive disorders.

For example, depressed adolescents with comorbid ADHD respond less well to SSRI treatment (Birmaher et al. 2000b; Emslie et al. 1998; Hamilton and Bridge 1999). For these patients, the ADHD should be treated first; if, after stabilization of the ADHD, the depressive symptoms continue, then an SSRI should be added (Hughes et al. 1999). However, this strategy has not been validated. Recently, an open study with bupropion suggested that this medication can be efficacious for the treatment of both the MDD and the ADHD (Daviss et al. 2001), although its effect on ADHD is not as impressive as that obtained with the stimulants (Conners et al. 1996).

Treatment of comorbid anxiety, which most often precedes depression, is essential insofar as it contributes to improvement and may predispose to future depressive episodes (Birmaher et al. 1996a, 1996b; Brent et al. 1998; Pine et al. 1998). Fortunately, similar pharmacotherapy and psychotherapy treatments found useful for the treatment of MDD also have been found beneficial for the treatment of anxiety disorders in youths (Kendall 1994; Research Units of Pediatric Psychopharmacology Anxiety Group 2001).

Suicidal ideation and behavior are common symptoms accompanying major depression and are more likely to occur in the face of comorbid disruptive behavior disorder, substance abuse, or the experience of trauma such as sexual abuse (Beautrais 2001; Gould et al. 1996). Assessment of suicidality, confiscation of any lethal agents (e.g., medications, firearms), and development of no-suicide contracts with the patient and family are essential components of the management of the suicidal, depressed patient (Brent et al. 1998; Shaffer and Pfeffer 2001). Patients who cannot agree to a no-suicide contract may require inpatient hospitalization. Treatment of the underlying depression may be necessary but not sufficient to prevent recurrent attempts, insofar as placebo-controlled medication trials in adults show greater improvement in depression associated with medication but equal rates of attempts and completions in medication plus placebo conditions (Khan et al. 2000). Other contributors to suicidality, such as sexual abuse, use of drugs and alcohol, conduct problems, impulsivity and aggression, personality disorders, and family discord, must be assessed and targeted (Beautrais 2000; Brent 1997).

Other comorbid conditions such as obsessive-compulsive, conduct, eating, and posttraumatic stress disorders also have been found to affect treatment response and need to be addressed for the successful treatment of depression in youths (Birmaher et al. 1996a, 1996b; Hughes et al. 1999).

Acute Treatment—Summary and Recommendations

Currently, the antidepressants of choice in treating youths with MDD are the SSRIs because they have been shown to be efficacious and safe for the treatment of MDD in children and adolescents, but further research on the other available antidepressants (e.g., bupropion, venlafaxine, nefazodone, mirtazapine) is needed. At standard doses (e.g., citalopram 20 mg/day; sertraline 50 mg/day; paroxetine 20 mg/day), child and adolescent patients should receive twice-a-day doses for at least 4–6 weeks before declaring lack of response to treatment (see "Treatment-Resistant Major Depressive Disorder" later in this chapter).

To plan an adequate treatment, the clinician should take into account factors such as the severity of the depression, subtype of depression (e.g., presence of psychosis, seasonal depression, bipolar depression), presence of comorbid disorders (e.g., ADHD, anxiety disorders, substance abuse, eating disorders, learning disabilities), treatment history, parental psychopathology, child's and parents' motivation toward treatment, clinician's motivation and expertise to perform the treatment, and presence of ongoing stressors (e.g., conflicts, abuse, academic difficulties).

The optimal pharmacological management of child and adolescent MDD involves some educative and supportive psychosocial interventions and management of daily problems. Education of the patient and family about the disease, nature of treatment, and prognosis is critical to engagement in treatment and enhancement of compliance (Brent et al. 1993).

The high degree of comorbidity, as well as the psychosocial and academic consequences of depression, emphasizes the importance of the use of adequate and carefully monitored polypharmacy treatments (e.g., SSRIs and stimulants for depressed patients with ADHD). Moreover, multimodal pharmacological and specific psychosocial (e.g., cognitive-behavioral therapy and interpersonal therapy) treatment approaches may be necessary (Birmaher et al. 1996a, 1996b; Hughes et al. 1999), especially in the face of family discord, a history of trauma, or "double depression."

Problems at school, academic issues, school refusal, abuse of drugs, exposure to negative events (e.g., abuse, conflict with parents), and peer issues must be addressed. For example, family discord is associated with slower recovery and greater chance of recurrence (Birmaher et al. 2000a; Emslie et al. 1998), and ongoing disappointments have been associated with chronic depression (Goodyer et al. 1998). Therefore, addressing family discord and improving patient coping skills are likely to improve outcome.

The high incidence of parental mental health problems and the fact that family psychopathology and conflicts have been associated with poor treatment response (Birmaher et al. 2000a; Brent et al. 1998) emphasize the need for evaluation and appropriate referral of parents and siblings of depressed youths.

Finally, evidence indicates that psychological "scars" affect youths even after the depression remits (e.g., poor self-esteem and social skills), which may need to be addressed with psychotherapy (Birmaher et al. 1996b, 2000a). Untreated depression may increase the likelihood of the development of personality disorders (Kasen et al. 2001; Lewinsohn et al. 1997).

Although it is beyond of the scope of this chapter, it is important to mention that specific psychotherapies (cognitive-behavioral therapy or interpersonal therapy) (Brent et al. 1997; Mufson et al. 1999) are also reasonable initial choices for the acute treatment of mild to moderate episodes of major depression in youths. Nevertheless, if patients are given psychotherapy alone, pharmacotherapy should be strongly considered to augment response if no improvement occurs by 4–6 weeks.

Continuation Therapy

To consolidate the response and prevent relapse of symptoms, the clinician should offer *all patients* continuation treatment for at least 6 months after complete symptom remission. Those who have shown difficulty achieving remission (≥3 months); have factors that have been associated with persistent depression, such as subsyndromal symptoms of depression, early onset, family history of recurrent depression, dysthymia, comorbid disorders, and suicidality; are exposed to stressors (e.g., family discord); or have a history of recurrent depression (American Academy of Child and Adolescent Psychiatry 1998; Birmaher et al. 1996a) should be treated longer (e.g., 1 year).

During this phase, patients are seen biweekly or monthly depending on the patient's clinical status, functioning, support systems, environmental stressors, motivation for treatment, and other psychiatric and medical disorders. The patient and his or her family should be taught to recognize early signs of relapse.

Pharmacotherapy Studies

Although continuation and maintenance strategies have not yet been adequately studied in children and adolescents, on the basis of studies with adults, during the continuation phase, the *antidepressants must be continued at the same dose used to attain remission of acute symptoms*, providing that there are no significant side effects or dose-related negative effects on the patient's compliance (American Psychiatric Association 2000). In adults, continuation pharmacotherapy treatment during this phase reduces the risk of relapse from 40%–60% to 10%–20%, with TCAs, SSRIs, and lithium carbonate having been found significantly more effective than placebo in preventing relapses (American Psychiatric Association 2000). Overall, more than 50% of the adult patients (American Psychiatric Association 2000) randomized to placebo relapsed during continuation trials, most within 3 months of having their medication discontinued.

At the end of the continuation phase, if the clinician decides that the antidepressants should be discontinued (see following section, "Maintenance Therapy"), it should be done gradually (e.g., 4 weeks) to avoid withdrawal effects such as sleep disturbance, irritability, and gastrointestinal symptoms, which may lead the clinician to misinterpret the need for continued medication treatment. Clinical practice has suggested that rapid discontinuation of antidepressants may precipitate a relapse or recurrence of depression. In children and adolescents, the treatment should be discontinued while they are on extended vacations rather than during the school year.

Follow-up studies of depressed youths and adults have shown that, despite successful acute psychotherapy or pharmacological treatment, the rate of relapse or recurrence at 6–12 months is about 40%–60%, particularly in those who discontinue treatment (Birmaher et al. 1996b, 2000a; Emslie et al. 1998). Naturalistic studies in children and adolescents, and controlled trials in adults, show that continuation medication and/or psychotherapy can reduce the relapse rates (Birmaher et al. 1996b; Emslie et al. 1998).

The patient and his or her family should be taught to recognize early signs of relapse. If relapse occurs, it should first be determined whether the patient was compliant. If the patient was not compliant, the antidepressant medication should be resumed. If the patient was compliant and had been previously responding to the medication (without significant side effects), the existence of ongoing stressors (e.g., conflict, abuse), comorbid psychiatric disorders (anxiety disorders; ADHD, inattentive or combined type; substance abuse; dysthymia; bipolar II disorder; eating disorder), and medical illnesses should be considered.

If relapse occurs, depending on the circumstances, an increase in the medication dose, change to other medication, augmentation strategies, or psychotherapy may be indicated. In studies of depressed adults, adding cognitive-behavioral therapy reduced the relapse rate compared with medication management alone (American Psychiatric Association 2000). However, this has not been studied in younger populations. For patients receiving only psychotherapy, adding medications and/or using new psychotherapeutic strategies should be considered.

Maintenance Therapy

After the patient has been asymptomatic for a period of approximately 6–12 months (continuation phase), the clinician must decide *who* should receive maintenance therapy, *which* therapy to use, and for *how long*.

The main goal of the maintenance phase is to prevent recurrences. This phase may extend from 1 year to much longer and typically is conducted at a visit frequency of 1–3 months depending on the patient's clinical status, functioning, support systems, environmental stressors, motivation for treatment, and other psychiatric and medical disorders.

Who Should Receive Maintenance Therapy?

The recommendation for maintenance therapy depends on several factors, such as severity of the present depressive episode (e.g., suicidality, psychosis, functional impairment), number and severity of prior depressive episodes, chronicity, comorbid disorders, family psychopathology, presence of support, patient and family willingness to adhere to the treatment program, and contraindications to treatment.

Factors associated with increased risk for recurrence in naturalistic studies of depressed children and adolescents may serve as guidance to the clinician to decide who needs maintenance treatment. These factors include history of depressive episodes, female sex, late onset, suicidality, double depression, subsyndromal symptoms, poor functioning, personality disorders, exposure to negative events (e.g., abuse, conflicts), and family history of recurrent depressive episodes (≥2 major depressive episodes) (Birmaher et al. 1996a, 1996b; Goodyer et al. 1998; Klein et al. 2001; Lewinsohn et al. 1999; Rao et al. 1999; Weissman et al. 1999).

Depressed *adults* (American Psychiatric Association 2000) who have only a single uncomplicated episode of depression, mild episodes, or lengthy intervals between episodes (e.g., 5 years) probably should not start maintenance treatment. Also, the consensus in adults is that patients with three or more episodes (especially if they occur in a short time and have deleterious consequences) and chronic depression should have maintenance treatment.

More controversy exists about whether to provide maintenance treatment to patients with two previous episodes. Overall, maintenance treatment has been recommended for adult depressed patients with two episodes who have one or more of the following criteria (Depression Guideline Panel 1993): 1) there is a family history of bipolar disorder or recurrent depression, 2) the first depressive episode was of early onset (before age 20), and 3) both episodes were severe or life threatening and occurred during the past 3 years. Given that depression in youths has a clinical presentation, sequelae, and a natural course similar to that in adults, the above-noted guidelines probably should be applied for youths with two previous major depressive episodes.

Which Therapy Should Be Used?

Practically, unless any contraindication (e.g., medication side effects) is present, the treatment that was efficacious in the induction of the remission of the acute episode should be used for maintenance therapy. However, patients who are maintained on only medications could be offered psychotherapy to help them cope with the "psychosocial scars" induced by the depression. Furthermore, many depressed youths live in environments charged with stressful situations, and their parents usually have psychiatric disorders, emphasizing the need for multimodal treatments.

In adults, pharmacological and psychosocial therapies have been efficacious in the prevention of depressive recurrences (American Psychiatric Association 2000). Because of the importance of developing preliminary maintenance treatment guidelines in children and adolescents with depressive disorders, pharmacological adult maintenance studies are briefly reviewed in the next subsection (see "How Long Should the Maintenance Phase Last?").

In selecting the medication for maintenance therapy, clinicians should consider the profile of side effects and the way these may affect the patient's compliance. For example, dry mouth, weight gain, increased sweating, sexual dysfunction, and polyuria (if patients are taking lithium) may be very troublesome and may induce discontinuation of treatment. In addition, in children and adolescents, the long-term consequences of using antidepressant medications (e.g., chronic inhibition of serotonin reuptake by SSRIs, tachycardia induced by TCAs) are not known.

Other factors, such as patients' embarrassment with friends, the idea of having "their minds controlled by a medication," taking medications as a sign of "weakness," and uncertainty about the risk of relapse in spite of doing well while taking medications, should be addressed with both patients and their parents.

How Long Should the Maintenance Phase Last?

Adult patients with second episodes who fulfill the criteria for maintenance therapy noted above should be maintained for several years (up to 5 years in adult studies) with the same dose of the antidepressant used to achieve clinical remission during the acute treatment phase. However, patients with three or more episodes and patients with second episodes associated with psychosis, severe impairment, or severe suicidality or that proved very difficult to treat should be considered for longer periods of or lifelong treatment (American Academy of Child and Adolescent Psychiatry 1998).

In summary, during the maintenance treatment phase (prevention of recurrences), pharmacological treatment has been found beneficial to prevent recurrences. Psychosocial (in particular, interpersonal therapy and cognitive-behavioral therapy) treatments also are efficacious, but in adults the current evidence is stronger for pharmacotherapy (American Psychiatric Association 2000). Also, it is not clear whether psychosocial treatments are efficacious to prevent recurrences for severe depressions. Psychosocial treatments may have promise in improving outcome in bipolar depression as well (Miklowitz et al. 1996). Psychotic, bipolar, and chronic depressions require use of medications.

TCAs, SSRIs, and lithium have been found efficacious for the prevention of depressive recurrences in adults (American Psychiatric Association 2000). However, given the above-noted advantages of the SSRIs and their efficacy in the acute treatment of MDD and dysthymia, this group is considered the first-choice medication. The antidepressant medication, unless it is not tolerated, should be continued at the full dose used to exert the initial therapeutic effect.

For children and adolescents with severe, chronic, or comorbid depression, history of trauma, or family discord, multimodal therapies are recommended. However, if antidepressant medications are used initially as monotherapy, psychosocial maintenance strategies should be implemented if residual social skills deficits or interpersonal conflicts are evident. The reduction of family stress, promotion of a supportive environment, and effective treatment of psychiatric disorders in parents and siblings also may help diminish the risk for recurrence.

Treatment-Resistant Major Depressive Disorder

Similar to the adult literature (American Psychiatric Association 2000), approximately 20%–30% of the youths with MDD have a partial (moderate response on the CGI Scale, presence of significant symptoms of MDD but not the full syndrome) or no response to treatment (e.g., Birmaher et al. 2000a). Patients with a partial response have a significantly higher rate of relapse during the first 6 months following therapy and have significantly more psychosocial, occupational, and medical problems (American Psychiatric Association 2000). Moreover, chronic depressions usually do not remit spontaneously and are not responsive to placebo (American Psychiatric Association 2000), indicating the need for aggressive treatment of these conditions.

The first step in the management of treatment-resistant depression is to establish the nonresponse. Several definitions of *nonresponse* have been used, including the presence of significant number of depressive symptoms, less than 50% improvement as measured by rating scales (e.g., the CDRS-R), and no change or worsening on the CGI Scale. Once it has been established that the patient has not responded, it is crucial to try to find the causes. The most common reasons for treatment failure are inappropriate diagnoses, inadequate drug dosage or length of drug trial, lack of compliance with treatment, comorbidity with other psychiatric (e.g., dysthymia, anxiety, ADHD, covered substance abuse, personality disorders) or medical illnesses (e.g., hypothyroidism), existence of bipolar depression, and exposure to chronic or severe life events (e.g., abuse, chronic conflicts) that require different modalities of therapy (American Psychiatric Association 2000; Brent et al. 1998; Emslie et al. 1998).

Very few pharmacological studies of children and adolescents with treatment-refractory depression have been done. After noncompliance with treatment has been ruled out, on the basis of the adult literature, the following strategies have been recommended: 1) optimizing the initial treatments, 2) switching to a different agent from the same group (e.g., one SSRI for another SSRI) or switching to a different agent from a different group (e.g., an SSRI to venlafaxine), 3) augmenting or combining treatments, 4) using electroconvulsive therapy (ECT), and 5) using other novel treatments (e.g., intravenous clomipramine, transcranial magnetic stimulation [TMS]) (for reviews, see American Academy of Child and Adolescent Psychiatry 1998; American

Psychiatric Association 2000; Martis and Janicak 2000; Thase and Rush 1997). All these strategies require implementation in a systematic fashion.

Psychoeducation with the patient and family is required to avoid the development of hopelessness both in the patient or family and in the clinician. Comparing these strategies with other treatments of medical disorders can be useful to help patients and their families understand the medication plan and to improve compliance and tolerance with treatment. The example of hypertension is appropriate: diuretics may be used alone or combined with other antihypertensives in different trials, according to response.

Optimizing Initial Treatments

Although few studies have evaluated the efficacy of optimizing the initial treatments, the initial treatment can be maximized by increasing the length of the trial or increasing the dose.

Extending the Initial Medication Trial

For patients with at least *partial response* after receiving a therapeutic dose of antidepressant for 6 weeks, the first and simplest strategy would be, if the patient's clinical and functional status allows, to extend the treatment for another 2–4 weeks (American Psychiatric Association 2000). This makes the most sense in the face of gradual and steady improvement.

Increasing the Dose

With partial or nonresponders, the dose can be increased and the patient observed for another 2–4 weeks (American Psychiatric Association 2000).

Switching Strategies

For patients who do not respond to a specific antidepressant medication or who do not tolerate its side effects, other antidepressants of the *same class* or *different classes* (e.g., venlafaxine for a patient treated with an SSRI) can be tried. In adults, about half of the SSRI nonresponders will respond to a switch to a second

SSRI (e.g., American Psychiatric Association 2000). The few adult studies published so far suggest that switching antidepressant classes is more efficacious than staying within the same class because of the probable heterogeneity in depression mechanisms. Also, severe depressions appear to respond better to antidepressants with both serotonergic and noradrenergic properties (e.g., venlafaxine) (Thase et al. 2001).

MAOIs have been found beneficial for adult patients who have not responded to other medications (American Psychiatric Association 2000; Thase and Rush 1997). An open study suggested that adolescents with depression who did not respond to TCAs responded to MAOIs (Ryan et al. 1988b). However, it is possible that these adolescents did not respond to TCAs because this group of medications is not efficacious for the treatment of pediatric MDD (Birmaher et al. 1996b). Because of the side-effect profile, and especially because of the need for dietary restrictions, these medications are not used frequently in adolescents.

Augmenting or Combining Treatments

The most common augmentation or combination strategies include adding lithium carbonate at therapeutic levels for 4 weeks, adding triiodothyronine (T_3) (25–50 µg/day), using stimulants, and combining an SSRI with a TCA (American Psychiatric Association 2000; Bauer et al. 2000). In adults, the addition of lithium to the antidepressants has increased the response rate (e.g., American Psychiatric Association 2000; Thase and Rush 1997). The interval before response to the augmentation with lithium has been reported from several days to 3 weeks (American Psychiatric Association 2000). After this period, the likelihood of observing improvement with lithium decreases.

In adolescents with MDD, an open study showed significant improvement of refractory depressive symptoms after augmentation of TCA treatment with lithium (Ryan et al. 1988a). Another open-label study, however, did not replicate this finding (Strober et al. 1992).

Case reports have suggested that adding stimulant medications or combining an SSRI with a TCA or bupropion also may be effective (American Psychiatric Association 2000), but these combinations must be done with caution because of the possibility of interactions (e.g., SSRIs and TCAs).

Additionally, in adults, the combination of antidepressants and psychotherapy (cognitive-behavioral therapy, interpersonal therapy) for patients with severe or treatment-resistant depression also has been useful (American Psychiatric Association 2000; Keller et al. 2000).

Electroconvulsive Therapy

ECT is one of the most efficacious treatments for adults with non-resistant (70% response) and resistant MDD (50% response) (American Psychiatric Association 2000). However, because of the invasiveness of this treatment, it remains the treatment of choice for only the most severe, incapacitating forms of resistant depression. No controlled studies have been reported in adolescents, but anecdotal reports have suggested that adolescents with refractory depression may respond to ECT without significant side effects (Rey and Walter 1997). Approximately 60% of the adult patients treated successfully with ECT tend to relapse after 6 months (American Psychiatric Association 2000). Therefore, they generally receive continuation and maintenance treatment with antidepressants, lithium, the combination of antidepressants and lithium, or maintenance ECT (American Psychiatric Association 2000; Sackeim et al. 2001). No maintenance ECT studies have been reported in depressed adolescents.

Other Treatments

Other innovative treatments such as intravenous clomipramine and TMS have been used in adults for the treatment of depression that has not responded to standard treatment. In adolescents, intravenous clomipramine has been shown to be efficacious for patients who have failed to respond to other antidepressant treatment (Sallee et al. 1997).

Some randomized controlled trials have shown that TMS seems efficacious and safe for the treatment of MDD in adults (with and without treatment-resistant depressions) (e.g., Martis and Janicak 2000). However, the use of TMS has not been standardized, and there is controversy regarding the methodology used in some studies.

Need for Further Research

Although the field has made some advances and we know that SSRIs are efficacious and safe for the acute treatment of childhood MDD, several areas need to be investigated. For example, do we treat an acute episode of depression with medication, psychotherapy, or both? Although currently under study, no extant head-to-head comparison of SSRIs and psychotherapy has been done in adolescents. What is the optimal time for continuation after achievement of symptom relief? Preliminary studies show that continuation treatment does prevent relapse, but the optimal period of coverage is not yet known (Birmaher et al. 1996b; Emslie et al. 1998).

As noted in the "Maintenance Therapy" section earlier in this chapter, some children and adolescents have a very chronic or recurrent course. In adults with similar types of depression, long-term treatment is recommended. Is this also the case for children or adolescents? Are there any long-term consequences of SSRI use in children and adolescents, whose brains are still developing during exposure?

Approximately 50%–60% of patients will respond to SSRIs, but a large proportion will not respond completely. We do not know the best approach for subjects who have not responded to acute treatment. In an ongoing National Institute of Mental Health–funded study of adolescents who failed to respond to an initial trial with an SSRI, the comparative efficacy of switching to another SSRI, to venlafaxine, or to either of these two strategies with cognitive-behavioral therapy is being compared. Are there clinical or biological indicators that may help to match treatment to patient profile? Perhaps pharmacogenetic markers may be able to identify nonresponders to SSRIs, guiding the clinician to seek alternative treatments.

The treatment of MDD and other comorbid psychiatric disorders in youths has not been rigorously evaluated with randomized clinical trials. This is particularly salient because it appears that MDD comorbid with ADHD may not respond as well to SSRIs as MDD without this comorbidity. Therefore, clinical trials with agents such as bupropion are indicated.

The proper treatment of depression in bipolar patients remains controversial. We do not know whether to treat a patient with periods of major depression and hypomania with an antidepressant or a mood stabilizer alone or with the combination of these two groups of medications. The treatment of depressed patients with psychosis or suicide attempters also has not been well addressed in the child literature; no controlled trials or even open-label studies are available to guide the clinician. Finally, although published guidelines and algorithms have been published (Birmaher et al. 1998; Hughes et al. 1999; Shaffer and Pfeffer 2001), these algorithms have not yet been evaluated.

References

Alderman J, Wolkow R, Chung M, et al: Sertraline treatment of children and adolescents with obsessive-compulsive disorder or depression: pharmacokinetics, tolerability, and efficacy. J Am Acad Child Adolesc Psychiatry 37:386–394, 1998

Ambrosini PJ, Wagner KD, Biederman J, et al: Multicenter open-label sertraline study in adolescent outpatients with major depression. J Am Acad Child Adolesc Psychiatry 38:566–572, 1999

American Academy of Child and Adolescent Psychiatry: Practice parameters for the assessment and treatment of children and adolescents with depressive disorder. J Am Acad Child Adolesc Psychiatry 37 (10 suppl):63S–83S, 1998

American Psychiatric Association: Practice guideline for the treatment of patients with bipolar disorder. Am J Psychiatry 41:1–35, 1994

American Psychiatric Association: Practice guideline for the treatment of patients with major depressive disorder (revision). Am J Psychiatry 157 (suppl):1–45, 2000

Amsterdam JD, Garcia-España F: Venlafaxine monotherapy in women with bipolar II and unipolar major depression. J Affect Disord 59: 225–229, 2000

Amsterdam JD, Garcia-España F, Fawcett J, et al: Efficacy and safety of fluoxetine in treating bipolar II major depressive episode. J Clin Psychopharmacol 18:435–440, 1998

Axelson D, Perel J, Rudolph G, et al: Sertraline pediatric/adolescent PK-PD parameters: dose/plasma level ranging for depression (abstract). Clin Pharmacol Ther 67:169, 2000a

Axelson D, Perel J, Rudolph G, et al: Significant differences in pharmacokinetics/dynamics of citalopram between adolescents and adults: implications for clinical dosing (abstract), in Proceedings of the 39th Annual Meeting of the American College of Neuropsychopharmacology, San Juan, Puerto Rico, 2000b, p 122

Bauer M, Bschor T, Kunz D, et al: Double-blind, placebo-controlled trial of the use of lithium to augment antidepressant medication in continuation treatment of unipolar major depression. Am J Psychiatry 157:1429–1435, 2000

Beautrais AL: Risk factors for suicide and attempted suicide among young people. Aust N Z J Psychiatry 34:420–436, 2000

Bernstein GA, Borchardt CM, Perwien AR, et al: Imipramine plus cognitive-behavioral therapy in the treatment of school refusal. J Am Acad Child Adolesc Psychiatry 39:276–283, 2000

Birmaher B, Ryan ND, Williamson D, et al: Childhood and adolescent depression: a review of the past 10 years—part I. J Am Acad Child Adolesc Psychiatry 35:1427–1439, 1996a

Birmaher B, Ryan ND, Williamson DE, et al: Childhood and adolescent depression: a review of the past 10 years—part II. J Am Acad Child Adolesc Psychiatry 35:1575–1583, 1996b

Birmaher B, Brent DA, Benson RS: Summary of the practice parameters for the assessment and treatment of children and adolescents with depressive disorders. American Academy of Child and Adolescent Psychiatry. J Am Acad Child Adolesc Psychiatry 37:1234–1238, 1998

Birmaher B, Brent DA, Kolko D, et al: Clinical outcome after short-term psychotherapy for adolescents with major depressive disorder. Arch Gen Psychiatry 57:29–36, 2000a

Birmaher B, McCafferty JP, Bellow KM, et al: Comorbid ADHD and disruptive behavior disorders as predictors of response in adolescents treated for major depression. Paper presented at the 153rd annual meeting of the American Psychiatric Association, Chicago, IL, May 13–18, 2000b

Brent DA: The aftercare of adolescents with deliberate self-harm. J Child Psychol Psychiatry 38:277–286, 1997

Brent DA, Poling K, McCain B, et al: A psychoeducational program for families of affectively ill children and adolescents. J Am Acad Child Adolesc Psychiatry 32:770–774, 1993

Brent DA, Holder D, Birmaher B, et al: A clinical psychotherapy trial for adolescent depression comparing cognitive, family, and supportive therapy. Arch Gen Psychiatry 54:877–885, 1997

Brent DA, Kolko D, Birmaher B, et al: Predictors of treatment efficacy in a clinical trial of three psychosocial treatments for adolescent depression. J Am Acad Child Adolesc Psychiatry 37:906–914, 1998

Brent DA, Baugher M, Birmaher B, et al: Compliance with recommendations to remove firearms by families participating in a clinical trial for adolescent depression. J Am Acad Child Adolesc Psychiatry 39: 1220–1226, 2000

Compton MT, Nemeroff CB: The treatment of bipolar depression. J Clin Psychiatry 61:57–67, 2000

Conners CK, Cast CD, Guiltieri CT, et al: Bupropion hydrochloride in attention deficit hyperactivity disorder. J Am Acad Child Adolesc Psychiatry 35:1314–1321, 1996

Daviss WB, Bentivoglio P, Racusin R, et al: Bupropion sustained release in adolescents with comorbid attention deficit hyperactivity. J Am Acad Child Adolesc Psychiatry 40:307–314, 2001

Depression Guideline Panel: Depression in Primary Care, Vol I: Treatment of Major Depression. Clinical Practice Guidelines. Rockville, MD, Agency for Health Care Policy and Research, 1993

Emslie G, Rush AJ, Weinberg AW, et al: A double-blind, randomized placebo-controlled trial of fluoxetine in depressed children and adolescents. Arch Gen Psychiatry 54:1031–1037, 1997

Emslie GJ, Rush AJ, Weinberg WA, et al: Fluoxetine in child and adolescent depression: acute and maintenance treatment. Depress Anxiety 7:32–39, 1998

Emslie GJ, Heiligenstein JH, Hoog SL, et al: Fluoxetine for acute treatment of depression in children and adolescents: a placebo controlled randomized clinical trial. Poster presented at the 39th annual meeting of the American College of Neuropsychopharmacology, San Juan, Puerto Rico, December 2000

Fava M, Rappe SM, Pava JA, et al: Relapse in patients on long-term fluoxetine treatment: response to increased fluoxetine dose. J Clin Psychiatry 56:52–55, 1995

Findling RL, Reed MD, Myers C, et al: Paroxetine pharmacokinetics in depressed children and adolescents. J Am Acad Child Adolesc Psychiatry 38:952–959, 1999

Geller B, Fox LW, Fletcher M: Effect of tricyclic antidepressants on switching to mania on the onset of bipolarity in depressed 6- to 12-year-olds. J Am Acad Child Adolesc Psychiatry 32:43–50, 1993

Goodyer IM, Herbert J, Altham PM: Adrenal, steroid secretion and major depression in 8- to 16-year-olds, III: influence of cortisol/DHEA ratio at presentation on subsequent rates of disappointing life events and persistent major depression. Psychol Med 28:265–273, 1998

Gould MS, Fisher P, Parides M: Psychosocial risk factors of child and adolescent completed suicide. Arch Gen Psychiatry 53:1155–1162, 1996

Hamilton JD, Bridge J: Outcome at 6 months of 50 adolescents with major depression treated in a health maintenance organization. J Am Acad Child Adolesc Psychiatry 38:1340–1346, 1999

Himmelhoch JM, Thase ME, Mallinger AG, et al: Tranylcypromine versus imipramine in anergic bipolar depression. Psychopharmacol Bull 148:910–916, 1991

Hughes CW, Emslie GJ, Crismon ML, et al: The Texas Childhood Medication Algorithm Project: report of the Texas Consensus Conference Panel on Medication Treatment of Childhood Major Depressive Disorder. J Am Acad Child Adolesc Psychiatry 38:1442–1454, 1999

Kapur S, Mieczkowski T, Mann JJ: Antidepressant medications and the relative risk of suicide attempt and suicide. JAMA 268:3441–3445, 1992

Kasen S, Cohen P, Skodol AE, et al: Childhood depression and adult personality disorder: alternative pathways of continuity. Arch Gen Psychiatry 58:231–236, 2001

Keller MB, McCullough JP, Klein DN, et al: A comparison of nefazodone, the cognitive behavioral-analysis system of psychotherapy, and their combination for the treatment of chronic depression: Multicenter Study. Randomized Controlled Trial. N Engl J Med 342:1462–1470, 2000

Keller MB, Ryan ND, Strober M, et al: Paroxetine for adolescent depression. J Am Acad Child Adolesc Psychiatry (in press)

Keller MB, Ryan ND, Strober M, et al: Efficacy of paroxetine in the treatment of adolescent major depression: a randomized, controlled study. J Am Acad Child Adolesc Psychiatry 40:762–772, 2001

Kendall PC: Treating anxiety disorders in children: results of a randomized clinical trial. J Consult Clin Psychol 62:100–110, 1994

Khan A, Warner HA, Brown WA: Symptom reduction and suicide risk in patients treated with placebo in antidepressant clinical trials: an analysis of the Food and Drug Administration database. Arch Gen Psychiatry 57:311–317, 2000

Klein DN, Lewinsohn PM, Seeley JR, et al: A family study of major depressive disorder in a community sample of adolescents. Arch Gen Psychiatry 58:13–20, 2001

Lake MB, Birmaher B, Wassick S, et al: Bleeding and selective serotonin reuptake inhibitors in childhood and adolescence. J Child Adolesc Psychopharmacol 10:35–38, 2000

Leonard HL, March J, Rickler KC, et al: Review of the pharmacology of the selective serotonin reuptake inhibitors in children and adolescents. J Am Acad Child Adolesc Psychiatry 36:725–736, 1997

Lewinsohn PM, Rohde P, Seeley JR, et al: Axis II psychopathology as a function of Axis I disorders. J Am Acad Child Adolesc Psychiatry 36:1752–1759, 1997

Lewinsohn PM, Allen NB, Seeley JR, et al: First onset versus recurrence of depression: differential processes of psychosocial risk. J Abnorm Psychol 108:483–489, 1999

Lewinsohn PM, Klein DN, Seeley JR: Bipolar disorder during adolescence and young adulthood in a community sample. Bipolar Disorders. 2:281–293, 2000

March JS, Biederman J, Wolkow R, et al: Sertraline in children and adolescents with obsessive-compulsive disorder: a multicenter randomized controlled trial. JAMA 280:1752–1756, 1998

Martis B, Janicak PG: Transcranial magnetic stimulation for major depression: therapeutic possibilities. International Drug Therapy Newsletter, July 1–10, 2000

Miklowitz DJ, Frank E, George EL: New psychosocial treatments for the outpatient management of bipolar disorder. Psychopharmacol Bull 32:613–621, 1996

Mufson L, Weissman MM, Moreau D, et al: Efficacy of interpersonal psychotherapy for depressed adolescents. Arch Gen Psychiatry 56:573–579, 1999

Mundo E, Walker M, Cate T, et al: The role of serotonin transporter protein gene in antidepressant-induced mania in bipolar disorder. Arch Gen Psychiatry 58:539–544, 2001

Pine DS, Cohen P, Gurley D, et al: The risk for early adulthood anxiety and depressive disorders in adolescents with anxiety and depressive disorders. Arch Gen Psychiatry 55:56–64, 1998

Pollock BG, Ferrell RE, Mulsant BH, et al: Allelic variation in the serotonin transporter promoter affects onset of paroxetine treatment response in late-life depression. Neuropsychopharmacology 23:587–590, 2000

Preskorn SH: Outpatient Management of Depression: A Guide for the Practitioner, 2nd Edition. Caddo, OK, Professional Communications, 1999

Rao U, Hammen C, Daley SE: Continuity of depression during the transition to adulthood: a 5-year longitudinal study of young women. J Am Acad Child Adolesc Psychiatry 38:908–915, 1999

Research Units of Pediatric Psychopharmacology Anxiety Group: Fluvoxamine for anxiety in children. N Engl J Med 344:1279–1285, 2001

Rey JM, Walter G: Half a century of ECT use in young people. Am J Psychiatry 154:595–602, 1997

Ryan N, Meyer V, Dachille S, et al: Lithium antidepressant augmentation in TCA-refractory depression in adolescents. J Am Acad Child Adolesc Psychiatry 27:371–376, 1988a

Ryan N, Puig-Antich J, Rabinovich H, et al: MAOIs in adolescent major depression unresponsive to tricyclic antidepressant. J Am Acad Child Adolesc Psychiatry 27:755–758, 1988b

Sackeim HA, Hasket RF, Mulsan BH, et al: Continuation pharmacotherapy in the prevention of relapse following electroconvulsive therapy: a randomized controlled trial. JAMA 285:1299–1307, 2001

Sallee FR, Vrindavanam NS, Deas-Nesmith D, et al: Pulse intravenous clomipramine for depressed adolescents: a double-blind, controlled trial. Am J Psychiatry 154:668–673, 1997

Shaffer D, Pfeffer C: Summary of the practice parameters for the assessment and treatment of children and adolescents with suicidal behavior. J Am Acad Child Adolesc Psychiatry 40:24S–56S, 2001

Simeon J, Dinicola V, Ferguson H, et al: Adolescent depression: a placebo-controlled fluoxetine treatment study and follow-up. Prog Neuropsychopharmacol Biol Psychiatry 14:791–795, 1990

Strober M, Carlson G: Bipolar illness in adolescents with major depression: clinical, genetic, and psychopharmacologic predictors in a three-to four-year prospective follow-up investigation. Arch Gen Psychiatry 39:549–555, 1982

Strober M, Freeman R, Rigali J, et al: The pharmacotherapy of depressive illness in adolescence, II: effects of lithium augmentation in nonresponders to imipramine. J Am Acad Child Adolesc Psychiatry 31:16–20, 1992

Swedo S, Allen AJ, Glod CA, et al: A controlled trial of light therapy for the treatment of pediatric seasonal affective disorder. J Am Acad Child Adolesc Psychiatry 36:816–821, 1997

Thase ME, Rush AJ: When at first you don't succeed: sequential strategies for antidepressant nonresponders. J Clin Psychiatry 58:23–29, 1997

Thase ME, Entsuah AR, Rudolph RL: Remission rates during treatment with venlafaxine or selective serotonin reuptake inhibitors. Br J Psychiatry 178:234–241, 2001

Weissman MM, Wolk S, Goldstein RB, et al: Depressed adolescents grown up. JAMA 281:1707–1713, 1999

Wilens TE, Wyatt D, Spencer TJ: Disentangling disinhibition. J Am Acad Child Adolesc Psychiatry 37:1225–1227, 1998

Chapter 4

Bipolar Disorder in Children and Adolescents

A Critical Review

Gabrielle A. Carlson, M.D.

Definitional Problems

When manic-depressive psychosis was originally defined in DSM-I (American Psychiatric Association 1952) and DSM-II (American Psychiatric Association 1968), confusion arose because patients who had only depressive episodes (now called *unipolar*) were included in this category. Since DSM-III (American Psychiatric Association 1980) reorganized the definition of mood disorders, *bipolar* was meant to clarify course (someone with bipolar disorder presumably has had at least one lifetime manic episode). However, being "bipolar" has come to be synonymous with "manic," and, ironically, it is difficult to know whether a patient who has bipolar disorder is having his or her lifetime characterized (i.e., no current problem but history of mania) or a current state identified and if that current state is a manic, depressive, hypomanic, or mixed episode. This chapter, although titled "Bipolar Disorder in Children and Adolescents," mainly concerns itself with mania in youths.

Other changes have occurred since DSM-III, including the definition of *episode*. This has alternated between 1 week and a "distinct period." Although DSM-IV (American Psychiatric Association 1994) re-identified the duration of "1 week" of symptoms for acute mania, subtypes called *rapid cycles* or ultrarapid cycles delineate much shorter periods. Hypomania, although formally defined as lasting 4 days, is generally characterized by symptoms of mild mania regardless of duration.

In the case of an adult who has lived many years before the onset of a mood disorder, distinguishing the subsequent course of mood disorder, regardless of the duration of manic or depressive symptoms, from the premorbid period may not be a problem. In children, however, this is problematic because premorbid is not a fixed entity. If the core symptoms of mania are dysregulated mood, excessive activity (mind and body), and inflated self-esteem, then the distinction between manic and nonmanic in children depends on developmental age. The range of activity level and attention span "allowed" for a 3-year-old is much greater than it is for a 10-year-old, which is why symptoms of attention-deficit/hyperactivity disorder (ADHD) have a developmental comparison built into the definition. Similarly, emotion regulation is developmentally mediated. Self-control over tears, anger, and excitement is expected to gradually increase through the preschool and school-age period. Finally, logical thinking increases with age such that formal thought disorder before age 7 years is more difficult to define (Caplan et al. 2000). Illogical thinking and formal thought disorder may occasionally occur even in healthy children through age 10. A 25-year-old convinced that he is a "superman" is grandiose. It is unclear whether a 5-year-old is.

Epidemiology

To understand the epidemiology of bipolar disorder, it is important to clarify whether one is considering lifetime rates of *bipolar disorder* or current rates of *acute mania*. Lifetime rates of bipolar I disorder (i.e., full-blown mania) in adults are 0.45% among men and 0.47% among women. The 1-year incidence was 0.36% (Kessler et al. 1997).

Two community studies of adolescents have been done: a small study of 150 adolescents aged 16 years (Carlson and Kashani 1988) and a large study in Oregon, the Oregon Adolescent Depression Project (OADP; Lewinsohn et al. 1995). In the former study, one subject was found to have had a lifetime episode of mania and of depression (0.06%), although rates of what we would now call hypomania and bipolar disorder not otherwise specified were 7% and 10%, respectively. Lewinsohn et al. (1995) reported lifetime rates of bipolar disorder of 0.95% in 14- to 18-year-olds. However, only two teenagers (0.1%) (gender not reported) had lifetime history of *mania*; the remainder reported lifetime hypomania (0.6%) with varying levels of depression severity (i.e., bipolar II disorder and cyclothymia [0.3%]). Basically, most subjects were depressed. The 1-year mania incidence was 0.13% (Lewinsohn et al. 2000). All of these rates were significantly lower than those seen in adults. Rates of 5.7% for at least 1 week of elated, expansive, or irritable mood, however, were similar to those reported in the Epidemiologic Catchment Area study for adults (Tohen and Goodwin 1995).

Because bipolar disorder often begins in adolescence and because several years may elapse before a person with bipolar disorder either seeks treatment or receives accurate diagnosis (McGlashan 1988), we might speculate that young people with subsyndromal mania or major depression would be at high risk to develop full-blown mania. However, a follow-up study of a subsample of the OADP subjects conducted when they were 24 years old showed that only three additional patients (annual incidence=0.08%) had developed acute mania (another three had developed hypomania). Only one of these had progressed from earlier hypomania; fewer than 1% of the adolescents with major depression had switched to mania. Subjects did not come from the 5.7% of the teenagers thought to have subsyndromal mania. Of those subjects who had a range of bipolar disorders (bipolar I and II disorder, cyclothymia), chronic or recurrent depression appeared to be the most persistent mood symptom (Lewinsohn et al. 2000). Thus, although in clinical samples acute, severe depression in youths often predicts a bipolar course (Goldberg et al. 2001), this may not be the case in nonclinical samples, and extrapolation from psychotically depressed inpatients to nonpsychotic outpatients should be done cautiously.

No reports on rates of mania in community studies of preteen mania/bipolar disorder have been published. In clinical samples, parents reported rates of a manic syndrome in 9% (Carlson et al.

1998) and 16% (Wozniak et al. 1995) of outpatients and 63% of in-patients (Carlson and Kelly 1998). Not surprisingly, when at least two informants are required to diagnose mania, rates decrease from 22% to 14% (Thuppal et al., submitted). Most of these patients have chronic mania or possibly a manic syndrome rather than classical manic depression.

In a follow-up study of children with ADHD, Biederman et al. (1996) found that 12% had acquired a lifetime manic episode over a 4-year period in contrast to 1.8% of the control subjects. In a follow-up study of 6- to 12-year-old boys who had been given diagnoses of minimal brain dysfunction, 13 of 75 (17%) met Schedule for Affective Disorders and Schizophrenia, Lifetime Version (SADS-L), criteria for lifetime bipolar spectrum disorder; however, only one of these had had mania; the remainder met Research Diagnostic Criteria for hypomania ($n=6$) or cyclo-thymia ($n=6$) (Carlson et al. 1999).

Comorbidity

Complicating the ascertainment of psychopathology and comor-bidity in mania is the fact that individual symptoms of mania characterize other psychiatric disorders, especially in children. The overlap of symptoms of hyperactivity and inattention with ADHD has been discussed (Milberger et al. 1995). However, "asso-ciated symptoms" in ADHD include sleep difficulty (power strug-gles getting to bed, arising early in the morning—both of which could be interpreted as "decreased need for sleep"), low frustra-tion tolerance, and emotional lability, which are indistinguish-able from irritability. Less publicized is that flight of ideas and rapid speech are seen in ADHD children with language disorders (Tannock and Schacher 1996). Irritability is a cardinal symptom of oppositional defiant disorder, depression, and anxiety accord-ing to DSM-III and DSM-IV. It is perhaps not surprising then that ADHD, oppositional defiant disorder, depression, and anxiety are the disorders most often found to co-occur with mania. In-deed, euphoria and grandiosity are, in fact, the only manic symp-toms unique to mania, and as pointed out at the beginning of this chapter, the developmental ramifications of these symptoms have yet to be delineated (Carlson 1998a).

In the United States, comorbidity has been associated with manic symptoms in adults (for review, see Hilty et al. 1999), in nonreferred populations (Kessler et al. 1994; Klein et al. 1996), and in children in association with depression, anxiety, oppositional defiant disorder, ADHD, and "organic" etiologies (e.g., closed head injury, frontal lobe syndromes), pervasive developmental disorder, and psychosis not otherwise specified (multidimensionally impaired) (for a review, see Carlson 1998b). Regardless of whether these comorbidities are spurious or true, mania or manic symptoms impose considerable additional impairment to the conditions with which they co-occur (Biederman et al. 1996; Carlson and Kelly 1998). Moreover, when externalizing disorders precede clear, psychotic bipolar disorder onset (which has been found in 21% of the bipolar subjects and 63% of those with adolescent onset), the 2-year outcome is significantly worse than it is for bipolar patients without childhood psychiatric symptoms (Carlson et al. 1999, 2000, in press). The combination, then, of a manic syndrome and disruptive behavior disorder confers clinically significant impairment and prognostic implications over and above what would occur if either condition occurred alone.

Interestingly, in other countries, early-onset bipolar disorder is very rare, and when it occurs, it lacks externalizing disorder comorbidity (Rasanen et al. 1998; Reddy et al. 1997; Srinath et al. 1998). One suspects that these countries are restricting their definition of bipolar disorder to the classical variety.

Obstetrical Complications

Pregnancy or obstetrical complications and developmental abnormalities have been explored in schizophrenia but until recently have not been the subject of research in bipolar disorder. Studies have associated obstetrical complications with early-onset bipolar disorder (Guth et al. 1993), severity and/or psychosis in bipolar disorder (Sigurdsson et al. 1999), and familiality in bipolar disorder (Kinney et al. 1993; Marcelis et al. 1998; van Os et al. 1995). These data suggest that the combination of genetic predisposition and early developmental insult may play a role in the development of affective disorders and perpetuation of impairment.

Neuroimaging Studies

Very few studies of structural brain differences between bipolar and nonbipolar children have been done. Botteron et al. (1995) compared age-matched nonbipolar control subjects with bipolar youths and found non–statistically significant differences in deep white matter hyperintensities, ventricular volumes (greater in bipolar patients), and cerebrum size (smaller in bipolar patients). In another study comparing schizophrenic, bipolar, and healthy 10- to 18-year-olds, Dasari and colleagues (1999) found no group differences between schizophrenic and bipolar youths, although both clinical groups had smaller intracranial and thalamic volumes and increased frontal and temporal lobe sulcal size when compared with the control subjects.

Castillo et al. (2000) used magnetic resonance spectroscopy in 10 bipolar and 10 nonbipolar control children aged 6–12 years. Glutamate-to-glutamine ratios in the frontal lobe and basal ganglia regions were increased, and lipid levels in the frontal lobes of the bipolar children were increased.

Delineating specific brain abnormalities in young people with bipolar disorder will require controlling for both developmental age and other comorbidities, which themselves produce abnormalities. It will be several years before this developing line of research provides definitive findings.

Phenomenology and Differential Diagnosis

Patients whose first episodes of mania or bipolar depression occur between ages 30 and 60 appear to have clearer episodes of mood disorder, have manias characterized by euphoria and irritability (rather than irritability alone), and are less likely to develop substance addiction (although they may engage in substance abuse as part of their acute episodes). Although psychosis occurs frequently, and can be quite severe, confusion with other disorders has not been a problem (Carlson et al. 1994). Response to lithium is generally considered good (Abou-Saleh 1993). The type of mania is termed *pure* rather than mixed, and one might call the kind of bipolar disorder *classical* or uncomplicated (Black et al. 1988).

Adolescent and young adult onset of bipolar disorder also may be classical, although more frequently these patients appear to have complicated forms of bipolar disorder. Traditionally, the diagnosis of mania was missed much more frequently in young patients than in bipolar patients with onset after age 30 (Joyce 1984). Severe psychosis used to be misdiagnosed as schizophrenia, but the tightening of schizophrenia criteria has lessened this (Carlson et al. 1994). Substance abuse both precipitates mania and may produce an organic psychosis difficult to differentiate from mania (Carlson et al. 1999; Goldberg et al. 1999). Comorbid and less psychotic forms of mania are confused with borderline personality disorder and "adolescent turmoil" (Weller et al. 1986).

Younger children with manic symptoms have never functioned well, have psychopathology that cuts across all disorders (anxiety, disruptive behavior, neuropsychiatric, cognitive, and developmental), and have mood symptoms that merge with other disorders, making episodes difficult to define. Although this form of "mania" and bipolar disorder is very different clinically from adult-onset, classical manic depression, it may relate to chronic "mixed" mania complicated by substance abuse and antisocial behavior in adults (Biederman et al. 2000b).

What is so different about mania delineated in children is the almost complete absence of classical manic-depressive illness, the co-occurrence of multiple other symptoms, and the presence of developmental problems as well (Faraone et al. 1997). If one examines the criteria for what had been called "organic mood disorder" in DSM-IIII-R (American Psychiatric Association 1987) (affective instability, e.g., marked shifts from normal mood to depression, irritability, or anxiety; recurrent outbursts of aggression or rage that are grossly out of proportion to any precipitating psychosocial stressors; marked impairment of social judgment, e.g., sexual indiscretions; marked apathy and indifference; and suspiciousness or paranoid ideation), one finds a perfect description of children who are receiving "bipolar" diagnoses. It is quite conceivable that the etiology of this condition will be different from the etiology of more classical, nonorganic manic-depressive illness.

Differential diagnosis of mania is also increasingly complicated by secondary agitation that occurs while taking multiple medications (Walkup and Labellarte 2001; Wilens et al. 1998). Activation and disinhibition may be difficult to distinguish from acute mania. Prospective study of children who become activated has not been done. Without such data, it is impossible to conclude whether the implications of this response are the same as they are with a switch into mania from a clinically depressed state. Practically speaking, it is sometimes necessary to hospitalize a child and discontinue all medications to really separate baseline disorder from secondary medication reaction.

Family Studies

Offspring of parents with bipolar disorder have 2.7 times greater risk for mental disorder and 4.0 times greater risk for developing a mood disorder than do offspring of parents with no mental disorder (LaPalme et al. 1997). This observation is so compelling that the trend in recent years has been to diagnose bipolar disorder in a child almost regardless of his or her symptoms if anyone in the family, no matter how distantly related, has a diagnosis of bipolar disorder. However, families of patients with early-onset bipolar disorder also have high rates of spectrum disorder (alcoholism, substance abuse, unipolar depression), antisocial personality, and comorbid bipolar disorder with ADHD, which are also heritable (Todd et al. 1996). Although there is a 9-fold increased risk for bipolar disorder in an offspring if he or she has one bipolar parent (1% unselected risk; 9% risk in offspring), the risk for Tourette's disorder if a parent has it is 25-fold, the risk for panic disorder is 12-fold, and the risk for ADHD is 5-fold (Nurnberger and Berrettini 1998). Thus, the notion that any bipolar disorder anywhere in the family negates any other psychiatric disorder or even that having a parent with bipolar disorder automatically makes the diagnosis in the child undoes the last 30 years of developing operational criteria to make a psychiatric diagnosis.

Two separate data sets suggest that there may be genetic subtypes of bipolar disorder. Duffy et al. (1998) found that offspring of lithium-responsive parents have fewer psychiatric symptoms and a more benign course than do offspring whose parents are not lithium responsive. Although the issue was approached differently, Biederman and colleagues (2000a) found that the highly comorbid youngsters with mania or manic syndrome seen in the Massachusetts General Psychopharmacology Clinic had family members with the same mood-dysregulated behavior rather than classical manic depression. That is, a child with mania and conduct disorder was significantly more likely to have family members with mania and antisocial disorders. The authors noted that when families were stratified into bipolar, antisocial, and other types, few differences emerged between the bipolar and the antisocial families (Faraone et al. 1998). The clinical implications of these data are significant. It means that when one obtains a family history of bipolar disorder, a distinction should be made between classical and complicated bipolar disorder. It also suggests that the treatment refractoriness of young manic children may be the same treatment refractoriness seen in aggressive children with conduct disorder.

Assessment

The National Institute of Mental Health Research Roundtable on Prepubertal Bipolar Disorder (2001) recommended two basic definitions of bipolar disorder: a narrow phenotype that adheres strictly to bipolar I and bipolar II criteria (with mania, hypomania, and depression clearly delineated) and a broader phenotype that "encompasses more heterogeneity, basically bipolar NOS [not otherwise specified], and includes children who do not quite meet criteria, but still are impaired by symptoms of mood instability" (p. 871). Children being labeled as "bipolar" on the basis of their mood-dysregulated behavior rarely meet formal criteria for either mania or bipolar disorder. Such children would more accurately be given a bipolar not otherwise specified diagnosis if they have some manic symptoms over and above ADHD symptoms but do not actually meet criteria. This would satisfy both accuracy and the need to assign a diagnosis for insurance purposes. It also would signal parents that we do not yet have a clear understanding of the relation between mood symptoms in their child and adult pure, mixed, or any bipolar disorder.

Interviews

The screening symptoms of mania—namely, euphoria and irritability—are not easy to assess. Euphoria is believed to be rare in children. A PubMed search found no articles on euphoria in children outside of a discussion of either substance abuse in teenagers or brain damage secondary to trauma. Parents of inpatient-referred 5- to 12-year-old children were asked about euphoria in their child in two ways. They were asked about "periods of 2 days or more when your child is abnormally cheerful much or all of the time." Only 8 of 171 parents (4.7%) agreed that their child was. They were also asked, "Does your child become very happy, silly, or giddy out of proportion to environmental situations?" Of the 130 parents, 37 (28.5%) said "yes." However, only 6 (4.6%) parents agreed that their child ever had a period in which they appeared to have a continuous feeling of extreme well-being. There was no relation between any of those parent-reported symptoms and subsequent corroboration by the child's inpatient nurse on the euphoria item of the Young Mania Rating Scale (Young et al. 1978), either after a week of hospitalization or after 2–3 weeks. In other words, cross-informant reliability was elusive (G. A. Carlson, unpublished data, June 2001).

Irritability is a problem to evaluate because of its frequency and lack of specificity rather than rarity. Parents of more than 25% of outpatients and 36% of inpatients described their child or adolescent as explosive and irritable often or very often (G. A. Carlson, unpublished data, June 2001). Because this symptom is a diagnostic criterion or associated feature in five different disorders (mania, depression, anxiety, oppositional defiant disorder, and ADHD), its presence signals severity and comorbidity. The most common reasons children and parents give for such explosions are being denied something they want, being frustrated when something does not work out, being provoked by peers, being surprised by a change in plans, and by transitioning from one activity to another. However, irritability has several dimensions. Some children explode quickly but calm down readily, and others do not explode often but are upset for hours. Children with pervasive developmental disorders can become explosive with change. Children with ADHD often become easily frustrated. Fatigue is an important precipitant of irritability. Children who develop insomnia while taking stimulants may become irritable secondary to inadequate sleep. In clinical practice, explosive episodes are increasingly being considered "rapid cycles." This remains to be proven.

Although structured interviews have helped to operationalize symptoms of the disorders they cover (for review, see Angold and Fisher 1999), most interviews do not ascertain information about conditions that previously were on Axis II or Axis III: pervasive developmental disorders, learning and language disorders, and medical and neurological disorders. Thus, children being evaluated for mania or bipolar disorder need to have those problems assessed separately. In addition, subsyndromal symptoms, which may be important to understanding psychopathology, often are not "counted." Anxious children, for instance, often have some symptoms of several anxiety disorders, are impaired by their anxiety, but do not quite "meet criteria" for one disorder. Finally, one of the reasons for the unreliability of structured interviews in children younger than 12 years is that the child may not really understand what is meant by certain terms. Concrete thinking is typical of children, and although more abstract thinking should be possible as the child approaches adolescence, children with learning disabilities and language disorders (and their parents) may endorse or deny symptoms that are absent or present. If the interview consists of having the child or parent only answer yes-or-no questions (without having them provide examples or, better still, describe the symptom before the interviewer tells them what to endorse), it will be impossible to know whether communication problems are present or the person has truly understood the concept being asked about.

Most clinicians do not have time to complete a structured interview on his or her patients. The point of a structured interview, however, is to cover all relevant symptoms and disorders. An interview conducted by an experienced and thorough clinician is successful because he or she understands a disorder well enough to recognize the import of symptoms described, ask for further elaboration, listen for examples the patient gives, and discern whether the examples are applicable. Kessler et al. (1997) reported that lay interviewers with structured interviews do not agree very well with clinicians in diagnosing mania. This may be part of the reason.

Rating Scales

Screening

The completion of rating scales by parents and teachers prior to evaluation is a time-honored tradition in child and adolescent psychiatry. To date, the Child Behavior Checklist (CBCL; Achenbach 1991) has been used as a screening instrument and appears to screen accurately for aggressive children with mood dysregulation, some of whom may have juvenile mania. Elevated scores (T scores > 67) on factor 3 (anxiety/depression), factor 6 (inattention), and factor 8 (aggression) is a consistent finding. These factors, and in some cases the delinquency factor, appear to peak regardless of whether the sample studied is from an outpatient department (Biederman et al. 1995; Carlson et al. 1998), inpatient service (Carlson and Kelly 1998), or research program (Geller et al. 1998). This is hardly surprising, however, because the "mania" samples were selected based on parent report of manic symptoms, and manic-depressive symptoms generally "load" on the anxiety/depression, aggression, inattention, and delinquency factors. Although these factors have distinguished groups of ADHD children from manic children, they have not been used in a general clinic prospectively to determine false-positive and false-negative cases.

We have used a DSM-IV–based rating scale—the Adolescent Symptom Inventory (Gadow and Sprafkin 1995)—to screen for cases of mania or bipolar disorder in a general outpatient clinic and found that when two sources of information (parent/teacher, parent/teen) reported manic symptoms, the child was more likely to meet criteria for either bipolar disorder or psychotic-like disorder (Thuppal et al., submitted). On an inpatient service in which the same rating scales were used, there was a severity gradient between children with "pure" disruptive behavior disorders, children with parent-reported manic symptoms, and children with parent- or teacher-reported manic symptoms. The latter children not only had the most severe symptoms but also were the most likely to be observed on the inpatient unit as having manic symptoms. Children with parent-reported manic symptoms alone had more heterogeneous psychiatric symptoms (Carlson 2001).

Ratings specifically of mania are limited and have not been examined developmentally.

The Young Mania Rating Scale (Young et al. 1978) has been used increasingly in drug studies of children (e.g., Kowatch et al. 2000), although surprisingly little work has been done on the instrument since the work of Fristad et al. (1992, 1995). The Young Mania Rating Scale is used in children as both a history-gathering and an interview measure, and it is not always clear which. Since younger children may not be able reliably to describe symptoms such as racing thoughts and flight of ideas, the therapist must meet with them to determine whether these and other symptoms are occurring. It is difficult to know what to make of a situation in which an informant or child says that his or her thoughts are racing, but no outward symptoms of this are present. Interviewing adolescents is less controversial, but the same considerations are present. Some items (e.g., insight) are simply not designed for children. Parents and children may differ in their responses to the presence or absence of certain symptoms. When this occurs, the clinician needs to meet with both simultaneously and come to a consensus about why they disagree.

Scales needed to assess mood disorder in children are not limited to mania. Just as interview questions are needed to ascertain depression, anxiety, ADHD, and aggression, rating scales also should be completed on those dimensions.

Treatment of Bipolar Disorder

Surprisingly, no randomized, double-blind, controlled studies of hospitalized children and adolescents with acute mania have been done. However, more information is available on lithium than on other mood stabilizers. Those data suggest that adolescents hospitalized with adolescent-onset acute mania have response rates of between 50% and 80% and that supplementation with sedating medication is common (Kafantaris et al. 1998; Strober et al. 1988, 1998). Naturalistic discontinuation of lithium (because of noncompliance) after stabilization resulted in relapse rates of 90% compared with 37.5% for those continuing lithium (Strober et al. 1990). A National Institute of Mental Health multisite study is currently examining this systematically. Children hospitalized with mania also respond to lithium (Varanka et al. 1988), but their comorbid disorders need separate attention (Carlson et al. 1992a, 1992b). More common are case series and open trials of mood stabilizers for acute mania (for review, see Davanzo and McCracken 2000). These studies, some of which were done in the 1970s and 1980s with "classical" adolescent manic patients, appeared to be promising in terms of their treatment efficacy for lithium. However, response to lithium was the reason, sometimes, that the diagnosis of manic-depression was made.

Open trials with divalproex sodium in hospitalized manic adolescents support its use (Deltito et al. 1998; Papatheodorou et al. 1995; West et al. 1994, 1995). Only case reports exist on carbamazepine (Craven and Murphy 2000; Hsu and Starzynsi 1986; Woolston 1999). These data are largely consistent with data from studies of hospitalized adults with classic mania. As in studies of adults, antipsychotic and/or antianxiety medications were frequently used adjunctively in subjects of these reports.

Electroconvulsive therapy has been used in treating refractory mania in two prepubertal children (Hill et al. 1997). Rey and Walter (1997) also summarized the literature on electroconvulsive therapy, including its successful use in mania in adolescents.

In outpatient samples with an assortment of bipolar and bipolar spectrum disorders, response rates are lower to all mood stabilizers (40%–50%), although the suggestion is that this response is similar to that in adults (Geller et al. 1998; Kowatch et al. 2000; Wagner et al., submitted). These data appear to be consistent with those from studies of adults with mixed mania or, similarly, mania spectrum disorders. Case series for atypical antipsychotics are encouraging, but more systematic data are needed (Frazier et al. 1999, 2001; Soutullo et al. 1999).

There are two studies of long-term mood stabilizer use. In a sophisticated chart review, Biederman et al. (1998) found that over a 2-year period, children with a clinically significant manic syndrome appeared to be functioning significantly better when mood stabilizers were continued. Delong and Aldershof (1987) collected 196 patients over the course of 10 years who were treated with lithium. They divided their sample into subgroups with either clear mood disorder or other disorders with manic-like symptoms. They determined response by whether patients continued taking lithium over a 10-month period. They also commented on whether relapse occurred on discontinuation. Not surprisingly, bipolar children and offspring of lithium-responsive parents had higher rates of response than did children with ADHD and affective symptoms or explosive behavior.

There are age-specific concerns about side effects of medications used to treat mania. For instance, the development of polycystic ovary disease (characterized by truncal obesity, hyperandrogenism, hyperinsulinemia, and lipid abnormalities) has been observed in only seizure patients taking divalproex as an anticonvulsant (Isojarvi et al. 1993, 1998). However, the fact that the subjects were young women who had taken the medication for several years has raised concern about the long-term implications of this drug for pubertal bipolar women. Certainly the prospects of chronic weight problems caused by any of the mood stabilizers or long-term renal effects of lithium might be expected to be more of an issue in people who have, by virtue of their young age at onset, been exposed to treatment longer.

Follow-Up

Considered a critical test of validity, follow-up as a way by which to clarify and differentiate outcomes has become complicated by different definitions of onset (episode onset or admission to study), recovery (how long without symptoms; symptomatic recovery or functional recovery), and sample characteristics (first vs. multiple episode, psychotic vs. nonpsychotic, comorbid/mixed/rapid cycling vs. "pure" manic). In studies of childhood mania, samples of youths with ADHD and comorbid mania have provided the major information.

A brief review of the data indicates that a tremendous difference exists between the outcomes of childhood or early adolescent mania and those of adolescent or adult onsets of more or less classical (even including comorbid) mania. Using an extremely liberal definition of recovery (2 weeks without manic symptoms in a highly comorbid sample of children with ADHD), Geller et al. (2000) found 6-month recoveries of less than 20%. This contrasts with a 90% recovery (2 months without symptoms) from pure mania and a 70% recovery from mixed mania in a hospitalized sample of adolescents with bipolar disorder (Strober et al. 1995). Keller et al. (1986) reported rates of recovery of about 80% in adults with pure mania and 55% in adults with mixed mania or rapid cycling from the National Collaborative Depression Study. However, some investigators have found a clear effect of age at onset on outcome (for review, see Suppes et al. 2000). Even adjusting for sex, education, and comorbidity, psychiatrically hospitalized psychotic bipolar patients with an age at onset before 19 years had an odds ratio of not remitting completely of 4.57 (1.57–13.20, $P<0.01$) (Carlson et al., in press). Reasons for these differences have yet to be clarified.

Summary

As the concept of bipolar disorder in adults has broadened and has come to include patients with chronic emotional dysregulation (Akiskal et al. 2000), it has been easier to find a diagnostic home for children with severe behavior problems that also include mood instability. Classic manic-depression is, in fact, rare before puberty. However, given the prognostic ramification of what Biederman et al. (2000b) called "a clinically significant manic syndrome," research interest in these children is both timely and necessary.

However, if psychiatry overbroadens bipolar disorder in the 1990s and 2000s as it did with schizophrenia in the 1950s and 1960s, and substitutes diagnosis on the basis of slippery criteria adherence and hearsay family histories as earlier psychiatrists used impressions and feelings to make diagnoses, we will have made little progress in the past 50 years.

References

Abou-Saleh MT: Who responds to prophylactic lithium therapy? Br J Psychiatry (suppl 21):20–26, 1993

Achenbach TM: Manual for the Child Behavior Checklist 4–18 and 1991 Profile. Burlington, University of Vermont, Department of Psychiatry, 1991

Akiskal HS, Bourgeois ML, Angst J, et al: Re-evaluating the prevalence of and diagnostic composition within the broad clinical spectrum of bipolar disorders. J Affect Disord 59(suppl):S5–S30, 2000

American Psychiatric Association: Diagnostic and Statistical Manual: Mental Disorders. Washington, DC, American Psychiatric Association, 1952

American Psychiatric Association: Diagnostic and Statistical Manual of Mental Disorders, 2nd Edition. Washington, DC, American Psychiatric Association, 1968

American Psychiatric Association: Diagnostic and Statistical Manual of Mental Disorders, 3rd Edition. Washington, DC, American Psychiatric Association, 1980

American Psychiatric Association: Diagnostic and Statistical Manual of Mental Disorders, 3rd Edition, Revised. Washington, DC, American Psychiatric Association, 1987

American Psychiatric Association: Diagnostic and Statistical Manual of Mental Disorders, 4th Edition. Washington, DC, American Psychiatric Association, 1994

Angold A, Fisher PW: Interviewer-based interviews, in Diagnostic Assessment in Child and Adolescent Psychopathology. Edited by Shaffer D, Lucas CP, Richters JE. New York, Guilford, 1999, pp 34–64

Biederman J, Wozniak J, Kiely K, et al: CBCL Clinical Scales discriminate prepubertal children with structured-interview-derived diagnosis of mania from those with ADHD. J Am Acad Child Adolesc Psychiatry 34:133–140, 1995

Biederman J, Faraone S, Mick E, et al: Attention-deficit hyperactivity disorder and juvenile mania: an overlooked comorbidity? J Am Acad Child Adolesc Psychiatry 35:997–1008, 1996

Biederman J, Mick E, Bostic JQ, et al: The naturalistic course of pharmacologic treatment of children with maniclike symptoms: a systematic chart review. J Clin Psychiatry 59:628–637, 1998

Biederman J, Faraone SV, Wozniak J, et al: Parsing the associations between bipolar, conduct, and substance use disorders: a familial risk analysis. Biol Psychiatry 48:1037–1044, 2000a

Biederman J, Mick E, Faraone SV, et al: Pediatric mania: a developmental subtype of bipolar disorder? Biol Psychiatry 48:458–466, 2000b

Black DW, Winokur G, Bell S, et al: Complicated mania: comorbidity and immediate outcome in the treatment of mania. Arch Gen Psychiatry 45:232–236, 1988

Botteron KN, Vannier MW, Geller B, et al: Preliminary study of magnetic resonance imaging characteristics in 8- to 16-year-olds with mania. J Am Acad Child Adolesc Psychiatry 34:742–749, 1995

Caplan R, Guthrie D, Tang B, et al: Thought disorder in childhood schizophrenia: replication and update of concept. J Am Acad Child Adolesc Psychiatry 39:771–778, 2000

Carlson GA: Juvenile mania vs ADHD. J Am Acad Child Adolesc Psychiatry 38:353–354, 1998a

Carlson GA: Bipolar disorder and attention deficit disorder-comorbidity or confusion. J Affect Disord 51:177–189, 1998b

Carlson GA: Informant interview differences in children hospitalized for manic symptoms. Presented at the International Society for Research in Child and Adolescent Psychopathology, Vancouver, BC, June 26–30, 2001

Carlson GA, Kashani JH: Manic symptoms in non-psychiatrically referred adolescents. J Affect Disord 15:219–226, 1988

Carlson GA, Kelly KL: Manic symptoms in psychiatrically hospitalized children—what do they mean? J Affect Disord 51:123–135, 1998

Carlson GA, Rapport MD, Pataki C, et al: Lithium in hospitalized children at 4 and 8 weeks: affective, behavioral and cognitive effects. J Child Psychol Psychiatry 33:411–425, 1992a

Carlson GA, Rapport MD, Pataki C, et al: The effects of methylphenidate and lithium on attention and activity level. J Am Acad Child Adolesc Psychiatry 31:262–270, 1992b

Carlson GA, Fennig S, Bromet EB: The confusion between bipolar disorder and schizophrenia in youth. J Am Acad Child Adolesc Psychiatry 33:453–460, 1994

Carlson GA, Loney J, Salisbury H, et al: Young referred boys with DICA-P manic symptoms vs. two comparison groups. J Affect Disord 51:113–121, 1998

Carlson GA, Bromet EJ, Lavelle J: Medication treatment in adolescents vs adults with psychotic mania. J Child Adolesc Psychopharmacol 9:221–231, 1999

Carlson GA, Bromet EJ, Sievers SB: Phenomenology and outcome of youth and adult onset subjects with psychotic mania. Am J Psychiatry 157:213–219, 2000

Carlson GA, Bromet EJ, Driessens C, et al: Age at onset, childhood psychopathology, and 2-year outcome in psychotic bipolar disorder. Am J Psychiatry (in press)

Castillo M, Kwock L, Courvoisie H, et al: Proton MR spectroscopy in children with bipolar affective disorder: preliminary observations. AJNR Am J Neuroradiol 21:832–838, 2000

Craven C, Murphy M: Carbamazepine treatment of bipolar disorder in an adolescent with cerebral palsy. J Am Acad Child Adolesc Psychiatry 39:680–681, 2000

Dasari M, Friedman L, Jesberger J, et al: A magnetic resonance imaging study of thalamic area in adolescent patients with either schizophrenia or bipolar disorder as compared to healthy controls. Psychiatry Res 91:155–162, 1999

Davanzo PA, McCracken JT: Mood stabilizers in the treatment of juvenile bipolar disorder. Child Adolesc Psychiatr Clin N Am 9:159–182, 2000

Delong GR, Aldershof AL: Long-term experience with lithium treatment in childhood; correlation with clinical diagnosis. J Am Acad Child Adolesc Psychiatry 26:389–394, 1987

Deltito AJ, Levitan J, Damore J, et al: Naturalistic experience with the use of divalproex sodium on an in-patient unit for adolescent psychiatric patients. Acta Psychiatr Scand 97:236–240, 1998

Duffy A, Alda M, Kutcher S, et al: Psychiatric symptoms and syndromes among adolescent children of parents with lithium-responsive or lithium-nonresponsive bipolar disorder. Am J Psychiatry 155:431–433, 1998

Faraone SV, Biederman J, Wozniak J, et al: Is comorbidity with ADHD a marker for juvenile-onset mania? J Am Acad Child Adolesc Psychiatry 36:1046–1055, 1997

Faraone SV, Biederman J, Mennin D, et al: Bipolar and antisocial disorders among relatives of ADHD children: parsing familial subtypes of illness. Am J Med Genet 81:108–116, 1998

Frazier JA, Meyer MC, Biederman J, et al: Risperidone treatment for juvenile bipolar disorder: a retrospective chart review. J Am Acad Child Adolesc Psychiatry 38:960–965, 1999

Frazier JA, Biederman J, Jacobs TG, et al: Olanzapine in the treatment of bipolar disorder in juveniles. J Child Adolesc Psychopharmacol 11:239–250, 2001

Fristad MA, Weller EB, Weller RA: The Mania Rating Scale: can it be used in children? A preliminary report. J Am Acad Child Adolesc Psychiatry 31:252–257, 1992

Fristad MA, Weller RA, Weller EB: The Mania Rating Scale (MRS): further reliability and validity studies with children. Ann Clin Psychiatry 7:127–132, 1995

Gadow KD, Sprafkin J: Adolescent Supplement to the Child Symptom Inventories Manual—3R. New York, Checkmate Plus, 1995

Geller B, Cooper TB, Sun K, et al: Double-blind and placebo-controlled study of lithium for adolescent bipolar disorders with secondary substance dependency. J Am Acad Child Adolesc Psychiatry 37:171–178, 1998

Geller B, Zimerman B, Williams M, et al: Six-month stability and outcome of a prepubertal and early adolescent bipolar disorder phenotype. J Child Adolesc Psychopharmacol 10:165–173, 2000

Goldberg JF, Garno JL, Leon AC, et al: A history of substance abuse complicates remission from acute mania in bipolar disorder. J Clin Psychiatry 60:733–740, 1999

Goldberg JF, Harrow M, Whiteside JE: Risk for bipolar Illness in patients initially hospitalized for unipolar depression. Am J Psychiatry 158:1265–1270, 2001

Guth C, Jones P, Murray R: Familial psychiatric illness and obstetric complications in early onset affective disorder: a case-control study. Br J Psychiatry 163:492–498, 1993

Hill MA, Courvoisie H, Dawkins K, et al: ECT for the treatment of intractable mania in two prepubertal male children. Convulsive Therapy 13:74–82, 1997

Hilty DM, Brady KT, Hales RE: A review of bipolar disorder among adults. Psychiatr Serv 50:201–213, 1999

Hsu LKG, Starzynski JM: Mania in adolescence. J Clin Psychiatry 47:596–599, 1986

Isojarvi JI, Laatikainen TJ, Pakarinen AJ, et al: Polycystic ovaries and hyperandrogenism in women taking valproate for epilepsy. N Engl J Med 329:1383–1388, 1993

Isojarvi JI, Rattya J, Myllyla W, et al: Valproate, lamotrigine, and insulin-mediated risks in women with epilepsy. Ann Neurol 43:446–451, 1998

Joyce PR: Age of onset in bipolar affective disorder and misdiagnosis as schizophrenia. Psychol Med 14:145–149, 1984

Kafantaris V, Coletti DJ, Dicker R, et al: Are childhood psychiatric histories of bipolar adolescents associated with family history, psychosis, and response to lithium treatment? J Affect Disord 51:153–164, 1998

Keller MB, Lavori PW, Coryell W, et al: Differential outcome of pure manic, mixed/cycling, and pure depressive episodes in patients with bipolar illness. JAMA 255:3138–3142, 1986

Kessler RC, McGonagle KA, Zhao S, et al: Lifetime and 12 month prevalence of DSM-III-R psychiatric disorders among persons aged 15–64 in the United States: results from the National Comorbidity Survey. Arch Gen Psychiatry 51:8–19, 1994

Kessler RC, Rubinow DR, Holmes C, et al: The epidemiology of DSM-III-R bipolar I disorder in a general population survey. Psychol Med 27:1079–1089, 1997

Kinney DK, Yurgelun-Todd DA, Levy DL, et al: Obstetrical complications in patients with bipolar disorder and their siblings. Psychiatry Res 48:47–56, 1993

Klein DN, Lewinsohn PM, Seeley JR: Hypomanic personality traits in a community sample of adolescents. J Affect Disord 38:135–143, 1996

Kowatch RA, Suppes T, Carmody TJ, et al: Effect size of lithium, divalproex sodium, and carbamazepine in children and adolescents with bipolar disorder. J Am Acad Child Adolesc Psychiatry 39:713–720, 2000

Lapalme M, Hodgins S, LaRoche C: Children of parents with bipolar disorder: a metaanalysis of risk for mental disorders. Can J Psychiatry 42:623–631, 1997

Lewinsohn PM, Klein DN, Seeley JR: Bipolar disorder in community sample of older adolescents: prevalence, phenomenology, comorbidity and course. J Am Acad Child Adolesc Psychiatry 34:454–463, 1995

Lewinsohn PM, Klein DN, Seeley JR: Bipolar disorder during adolescence and young adulthood in a community sample. Bipolar Disorders 2(3 pt 2):281–293, 2000

Marcelis M, van Os J, Sham P, et al: Obstetric complications and familial morbid risk of psychiatric disorders. Am J Med Genet 81:29–36, 1998

McGlashan TH: Adolescent versus adult onset of mania. Am J Psychiatry 145:221–223, 1988

Milberger S, Biederman J, Faraone SV, et al: Attention deficit hyperactivity disorder and comorbid disorders: issues of overlapping symptoms. Am J Psychiatry 152:1793–1799, 1995

National Institute of Mental Health Research Roundtable on Prepubertal Bipolar Disorder. J Am Acad Child Adolesc Psychiatry 40(8):871–878, 2001

Nurnberger J, Berrettini W: Psychiatric Genetics. London, Chapman & Hall, 1998

Papatheodorou G, Kutcher SP, Katic M, et al: The efficacy and safety of divalproex sodium in the treatment of acute mania in adolescents and young adults: an open clinical trial. J Clin Psychopharmacol 15:110–116, 1995

Rasanen P, Tiihonen J, Hakko H: The incidence and onset-age of hospitalized bipolar affective disorder in Finland. J Affect Disord 48:63–68, 1998

Reddy YC, Girimaji S, Srinath S: Clinical profile of mania in children and adolescents from the Indian subcontinent. Can J Psychiatry 42:841–846, 1997

Rey JM, Walter G: Half a century of ECT use in young people. Am J Psychiatry 154:595–602, 1997

Sigurdsson E, Fombonne E, Sayal K, et al: Neurodevelopmental antecedents of early onset bipolar affective disorder. Br J Psychiatry 174:121–127, 1999

Soutullo CA, Sorter MT, Foster KD, et al: Olanzapine in the treatment of adolescent acute mania: a report of seven cases. J Affect Disord 53:279–283, 1999

Srinath S, Janardhan Reddy YC, Girimaji SR, et al: A prospective study of bipolar disorder in children and adolescents from India. Acta Psychiatr Scand 98:437–442, 1998

Strober M, Morrell W, Burroughs J, et al: A family study of bipolar I disorder in adolescence. J Affect Disord 15:255–268, 1988

Strober M, Morrell W, Lampert C, et al: Relapse following discontinuation of lithium maintenance therapy in adolescents with bipolar I illness: a naturalistic study. Am J Psychiatry 147:457–461, 1990

Strober M, Schmidt-Lackner S, Freeman R, et al: Recovery and relapse in adolescents with bipolar affective illness: a five-year naturalistic, prospective follow-up. J Am Acad Child Adolesc Psychiatry 34:724–731, 1995

Strober M, DeAntonio M, Schmidt-Lackner S, et al: Early childhood attention deficit hyperactivity disorder predicts poorer response to acute lithium therapy in adolescent mania. J Affect Disord 51:145–151, 1998

Suppes T, Dennehy EB, Gibbons EW: The longitudinal course of bipolar disorder. J Clin Psychiatry 61 (suppl 9):23–30, 2000

Tannock R, Schacher R: Executive dysfunction as an underlying mechanism of behavior and language problems in attention-deficit/hyperactivity disorder, in Language, Learning, and Behavior Disorders: Developmental, Biological, and Clinical Perspectives. Edited by Beitchman JH, Cohen NJ, Konstantareas MM, et al. New York, Cambridge University Press, 1996

Todd RD, Geller B, Neuman R, et al: Increased prevalence of alcoholism in relatives of depressed and bipolar children. J Am Acad Child Adolesc Psychiatry 35:716–724, 1996

Tohen M, Goodwin FK: Epidemiology of bipolar disorder, in Textbook in Psychiatric Epidemiology. Edited by Tsuang MT, Tohen M, Zahner GEP. New York, Wiley-Liss, 1995, pp 301–316

van Os J, Takei N, Castle DJ, et al: Premorbid abnormalities in mania, schizomania, acute schizophrenia, and chronic schizophrenia. Soc Psychiatry Psychiatr Epidemiol 30:274–278, 1995

Varanka TM, Weller RA, Weller EB, et al: Lithium treatment of manic episodes with psychotic features in prepubertal children. Am J Psychiatry 145:1557–1559, 1988

Walkup J, Labellarte M: Complications of SSRI treatment. J Child Adolesc Psychopharmacol 11:1–4, 2001

Weller RA, Weller EB, Tucker SG, et al: Mania in prepubertal children: has it been underdiagnosed? J Affect Disord 11:151–154, 1986

West SA, Keck PE Jr, McElroy SL, et al: Open trial of valproate in the treatment of adolescent mania. J Child Adolesc Psychopharmacol 4:263–267, 1994

West SA, Keck PE Jr, McElroy SL: Oral loading doses in the valproate treatment of adolescents with mixed bipolar disorder. J Child Adolesc Psychopharmacol 5:225–231, 1995

Wilens TE, Wyatt D, Spencer TJ: Disentangling disinhibition. J Am Acad Child Adolesc Psychiatry 37:1225–1227, 1998

Woolston JL: Case study: carbamazepine treatment of juvenile-onset bipolar disorder. J Am Acad Child Adolesc Psychiatry 38:335–338, 1999

Wozniak J, Biederman J, Kiely K, et al: Mania-like symptoms suggestive of childhood-onset bipolar disorder in clinically referred children. J Am Acad Child Adolesc Psychiatry 34:867–876, 1995

Young RC, Biggs JT, Ziegler VE, et al: A rating scale for mania: reliability, validity and sensitivity. Br J Psychiatry 133:429–435, 1978

Chapter 5

Suicide and Suicidal Behavior in Children and Adolescents

David Shaffer, F.R.C.P.(Lond), F.R.C.Psych.(Lond)
Ted Greenberg, M.P.H.

The general tenor of the Review of Psychiatry Series is to emphasize a "how-to" aspect of diagnosis, treatment, and prevention (Oldham and Riba 1998). Suicide, which nearly always occurs in the context of a preexisting psychiatric disturbance, presents challenges and opportunities for clinicians. A well-based strategy for clinical diagnosis and treatment is an essential component. Although we are still some way from well-tested management algorithms for suicide attempters, there have been substantial advances in our knowledge of *which* teens commit suicide and ever-increasing information on effective and ineffective treatments. Meanwhile, the youth suicide rate has been declining each year, and it seems likely that this is the result of better treatment of more depressed teenagers. For the first time, preventing youth suicide has become a tangible goal.

Suicidality includes suicidal ideation, suicide attempts, and suicide completions, which are imperfectly nested within one another. It is not possible to attempt or commit suicide without thinking about it, but only one in three ideators will ever attempt suicide. Up to 40% of the teenagers who commit suicide have made a prior attempt (for a summary, see Groholt et al. 1997), but in the United States, 400 teenaged boys and 4,000 teenaged girls will attempt suicide for every boy or girl who commits suicide

(Centers for Disease Control and Prevention 2000; National Center for Health Statistics 2001a). Many suicides occur under circumstances in which timely discovery was possible and death can reasonably be seen as an "attempt gone wrong." Finally, after standardizing for gender, no clear differences between attempters and completers have ever been identified other than choice of method. There is, in other words, an almost inextricable net of similarity and difference. And for most clinical purposes, it is sensible, if frustrating, to assume that the most minor manifestations of suicidality could presage a tragic outcome, although it is highly unlikely that they will.

Epidemiology

Suicidal Ideation

The Youth Risk Behavior Survey (YRBS) conducted by the Centers for Disease Control and Prevention (CDC) obtains information about ideation from between 12,000 and 16,000 school attendees aged 14–17 years every 2 years. Since 1991, the survey has recorded endorsements of the question "Have you seriously considered suicide within the last year?" ranging between 25% and 37% among girls and 14% and 21% among boys (Centers for Disease Control and Prevention 2000). Of the ideators, 75% had also formulated a suicide plan.

In regular high-school students, both ideation and attempts were more common in Hispanics than in whites, although in a separate survey of alternative high schools (Centers for Disease Control and Prevention 1999), the highest rates were found in whites. Although these rates of ideation seem high, similar rates have been reported in samples of 15-year-olds (Garrison et al. 1991b; Reinherz et al. 1995), in 12- to 14-year-old urban high-school students (Kandel et al. 1991), and in Canadian teenagers (Dubow 1989). Community-based studies indicated that approximately half of all teenaged ideators had ideated only once, whereas 10% had ideated more than three times in the past 6 months (Choquet and Menke 1989; Reifman and Windle 1995). Ideation is nearly always episodic, and Garrison et al. (1991a), in a longitudinal study of 12- to 16-year-olds, found relatively weak correlations of ideation from one year to another. It is not known whether demographic or clinical differences differentiate frequent and infrequent ideators.

Secular Change

The rates of ideation as recorded in the YRBS declined from 21% in males and 29% in females in 1991 to 15% and 22%, respectively, in 1999.

Suicide Attempts

In 1999, the YRBS reported that 11% of the female and 6% of the male high-school students had made an attempt in the previous year (1.8:1). The peak incidence was among 15- to 16-year-olds. The rates were much higher in alternative schools (20% in males and 12% in females). Between 2% and 3% of the teenagers received medical attention for their attempt. The female-to-male ratio in community studies is much lower than that found in clinic settings, where it ranges from 3:1 to 7:1 (Chung et al. 1987; Sellar et al. 1990). The higher proportion of females found in clinical settings could reflect the female method preference for ingestion of drugs, which may be more likely to lead to medical attention than other failed methods.

Secular Change

In the United States, the suicide attempt rate since 1990 has remained steady at about 11% for females and 4% for males (Centers for Disease Control and Prevention 2000). It is difficult to compare these observations with reports of increasing incidence rates in Europe over the same time (Hawton et al. 1998, 2000a; Schmidtkte et al. 1996), which are based on clinical rather than community samples.

Method

In general population samples, the methods used by most girls are ingestion (55%) and skin cutting (31%). Attempt methods are more varied among males: 25% skin cutting, 20% ingestion, 15% firearms, and 11% hanging (Lewinsohn et al. 1996). In both North

American and Western European *clinics,* most attempts are by overdose, nearly always of a nonnarcotic analgesic or psychotropic drug (Michel et al. 2000; Spirito et al. 1989; Velez and Cohen 1988).

Repeat Attempts

From 12% to 30% of adolescent suicide attempters seen in clinics report having made a prior attempt (Hawton et al. 1982a; Rohn et al. 1977; White 1974). In a prospective, community-based sample, the repeat incidence rate was 10% over 2 years (Lewinsohn et al. 1994); most repeats took place within 3 months of the initial attempt. Repeat attempts are more common in males; in teenagers with a history of substance abuse, psychosis, and depressive symptomatology (Gispert et al. 1987; Hawton et al. 1993, 1999); in those living away from biological parents; and in those with poor peer relationships (Goldacre and Hawton 1985; Pfeffer et al. 1991; Stanley and Barter 1970; Vajda and Steinbeck 2000).

Later Suicide

Prospective studies of clinic cases have shown that between 0.1% and 11% of adolescent suicide attempters will eventually commit suicide (Goldacre and Hawton 1985; Motto 1984; Otto 1972; for a review, see Spirito et al. 1989). The likelihood of later suicide is greater in older teenagers, in males, and in those who have been hospitalized. In Otto's (1972) study, 70% of the attempters who ultimately completed suicide died by methods similar to those used in their initial attempt, and the remainder used a more lethal method.

Completed Suicide

In most developed countries, suicide is the second leading cause of death, exceeded only by accidents.

Age

The incidence of suicide is very low before puberty (see Figure 5–1), is steady through the teenaged years in girls, but increases rapidly in boys after age 15, reaching a peak in the early 20s.

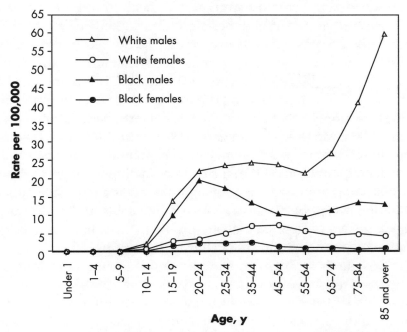

Figure 5–1. Suicide rates per 100,000 living population (all ages, 1999). *Source.* National Center for Health Statistics 2001a.

Sex

In most countries, completed suicides are more common in males. But in a few countries, notably China and India, the suicide rate is higher among females (National Crime Records Bureau 2001; World Health Organization 2000). It is not known whether the sex difference in these countries is due to some unique cultural factor or to the treatability of the preferred suicide attempt method.

Race/Ethnicity

The suicide rate in the United States has, for many years, been considerably higher in whites than in nonwhites in all sex and age groups (see Figure 5–1). In the mid-1980s, the suicide rate among African American male teenagers began to increase precipitously. Several years later, it started to decrease. This decrease took place several years after the decline in whites (see Figure 5–2). Declines have continued in both racial/ethnic groups, and teenage white rates remain marginally higher, although not to the same extent as in earlier generations. Black-white differences in the United States have been variously attributed to religiosity (Neeleman et al. 1998), more effective social support systems (Bush 1976; Gibbs and Martin 1964; May 1987; Neeleman and Wessely 1999), and reporting differences. African American suicides are more likely to be listed as "undetermined" (Mohler and Earls 2001; Monk and Warshauer 1978), but the size of this reporting difference is not sufficient to explain the discrepancy in incidence. Variations in the suicide rates in different racial/ethnic or cultural groups, nations, or geographic areas are the rule rather than the exception. They are remarkably stable and poorly understood. It may be that they are driven by imitation or identification operating within culturally similar groups.

Despite these differences in rates, no evidence indicates that the characteristics of suicides (i.e., types of psychiatric diagnoses, familial incidence, and precipitating stresses) differ by race/ethnicity. Indeed, they are similar in countries as different from the United States (Shaffer et al. 1996) as Finland (Marttunen et al. 1991, 1993), India (Vijayakumar and Rajkumar 1999), and both Han Chinese and aboriginal Formosans in Taiwan (Cheng 1995).

Season

Suicide is most common during the spring months in both the Northern and Southern Hemispheres (Chew and McCleary 1995; Flisher et al. 1997; Lester 1979), with a second peak in autumn (Hakko et al. 1998; Kevan 1980; Meares et al. 1981). However, within the last 20 years, seasonal variation has shown a marked flattening (Ho et al. 1997; Parker et al. 2001; Rihmer et al. 1998; Yip et al. 1998, 2000).

Similar seasonal peaks in hypomanic behavior occur among individuals with bipolar illness (Eastwood and Peter 1988; Goodwin and Jamison 1990; Silverstone et al. 1995; Szabo and Blanche 1995). Among patients with bipolar illness, suicide is most common at the time of mood shifts, and there might be an association between the two phenomena. The recent flattening of seasonal variation would be compatible with a reduction in the number of individuals with uncontrolled bipolar illness.

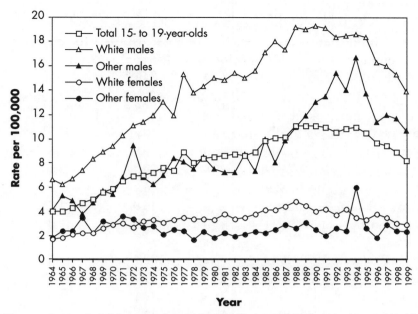

Figure 5–2. Suicide rates per 100,000 living population (ages 15–19, 1964–1999).

Source. National Center for Health Statistics 2001a (1999 data are preliminary).

Change in Incidence

In the United States and in many other countries, the incidence of youth suicide has changed considerably over the past 40 years (Figure 5–2). Between the mid-1960s and the mid-1980s, United States suicides in male teenagers increased more than threefold (National Center for Health Statistics 2000), with similar increases being reported in many other countries (Lynskey et al. 2000; Mc-Clure 2000; World Health Organization 2000). However, after 1990, the trend was reversed. Between 1990 and 2000, the suicide rate in boys aged 15–24 declined by 21.7% in the United States and by 27.8% in Australia. Between 1990 and 1999 (the most recently reported year in many countries), the suicide rate declined by 11.5% in Hungary and 19.0% in the United Kingdom. Sweden experienced a decline of 41.5% between 1989 and 1998 (Table 5–1).

Several explanations were advanced for the *increase.* They included demographic change, with an increase in the density of the adolescent population (Holinger et al. 1988), and (in the pop-

Table 5–1. Youth suicide among males, aged 15 to 24 years, in selected countries during the 1990s

Country	Period	Mean rate Time 1[†]	Rate Time 2	Time 1–Time 2
Sweden[a]	1989/1998	18.3	10.7	−41.5%
Australia[b]	1990/2000	26.3	19.0	−27.8%
Austria[c]	1990/1999	26.4	20.3	−23.1%
Finland[d]	1990/1999	47.0	36.3	−22.8%
United States[e]	1990/2000	21.6	16.9[‡]	−21.7%
England and Wales[f]	1990/1999	11.0	8.9	−19.0%
New Zealand[g]	1990/1999	37.2	30.3[‡]	−18.5%
Canada[h]	1989/1998	24.7	21.9	−11.5%
Hungary[c]	1990/1999	21.6	19.1	−11.5%
France[c]	1989/1997	14.8	13.4	−9.5%
Bulgaria[c]	1990/1999	12.4	12.0	−3.2%
Japan[c]	1989/1997	10.6	11.3	6.6%
Poland[c]	1990/1999	15.3	21.7	41.8%
Ireland[i]	1990/2000	14.2	26.2	84.5%

[†]Mean annual rate per 100,000 for 3 years preceding end of period.
[‡]Preliminary.
Source. [a]Statistics Sweden 2001; [b]Australian Bureau of Statistics 2001; [c]World Health Organization 1987–1995, 2001; [d]Statistics Finland 2001; [e]National Center for Health Statistics 1999, 2001b; [f]United Kingdom Office for National Statistics 2000; [g]New Zealand Health Informationa Service 2001; [h]Statistics Canada 2001; [i]Central Statistics Office of Ireland 2001.

ular media) rising divorce and maternal employment rates, the prevalence of suicide as a theme in popular music, and demonic themes in role-playing games (see Shaffer et al. 1988). Evidence for the demographic explanations was at best ecological, and none of these suggestions took into account what had been learned from psychological autopsy studies (i.e., that family composition varies little between suicide completers and control subjects and that most people who commit suicide have a psychiatric disorder at the time of death). Between the mid-1960s and the mid-1980s, the use of drugs and alcohol markedly increased. This is a plausible link for two reasons: 1) alcohol and substance abuse are important risk factors for suicide in adults and adolescents (Murphy and Robins 1967; Murphy and Wetzel 1990; Renaud et al. 1999; Robins et al. 1959; Shaffer et al. 1996), and 2) the relation between alcohol and suicidality seems to be more marked in males than in females, and the marked increase in teenage suicide rates was confined to males.

However the subsequent *decrease* in the suicide rate between 1988 and 2000 cannot be explained by less exposure to drugs and alcohol because usage rates were steady or increased slightly during that period (Centers for Disease Control and Prevention 2000; United Kingdom Office for National Statistics 2000). This period coincides with a very substantial increase in the prescribing of antidepressants for the general teenage population (Isacsson et al. 1997; Ohberg et al. 1998; Olfson et al. 1998; Rihmer et al. 1998; Rushton and Whitmire 2001; Safer 1997). Although no randomized controlled trials of selective serotonin reuptake inhibitor (SSRI) antidepressants showed an antisuicidal effect in teenagers, studies in adults have confirmed this effect (Verkes et al. 1998a). Other support for this explanation of the declining suicide rate has been reported by Isacsson et al. (1996, 1997), who calculated the population prevalence of SSRI-treated adult depression in Sweden and found that this was considerably higher than the rate of SSRI-positive autopsies among persons who committed suicide, suggesting that they were significantly undertreated. Finally, evidence from several countries suggests that the seasonal variations in suicide, probably a marker of bipolarity, have declined recently (Hakko et al. 1998; Rihmer et al. 1998; Yip et al. 1998, 2000). One might expect such a finding if individuals with bipolar disorder—at risk for suicide—were now being given more effective treatment.

Clinical Manifestations

Suicidal Ideation

Definition

Suicidal ideation can range from a fleeting vengeful or despairing thought experienced during a moment of anger, frustration, or loss by a youngster who, having been found out in some misdeed, is dreading a disciplinary response to a quiet, silent, and planned preoccupation in a depressed individual who feels hopeless to an all-consuming, ruminative preoccupation in an individual who has developed akathisia from a neuroleptic or an SSRI.

The content and form of suicidal ideas generally are understudied and often go unexplained. We have a very poor understanding of the relative importance of cognitive distortions, behavioral dyscontrol, and ease of access to method in transforming suicidal thoughts into behavior.

The YRBS found that most ideators made suicide plans when they thought about suicide. Suicide is probably most often thought of as a complete action rather than as an abstraction, and the time-honored clinical inquiry about planning is almost certainly a poor measure of serious intent. In their analysis of YRBS data, Simon and Crosby (2000) found that nonplanner ideators were just as likely to attempt suicide as were planners and that the nonplanners carried additional risk factors.

Associated Psychopathology

Although adolescent suicidal ideation usually is associated with psychopathology, in a study by Gould et al. (1998), approximately one-third of the 1,285 randomly selected children aged 9–17 had no associated psychopathology. Ideation was approximately six or seven times more common in high-school students with a mood, anxiety, conduct, or oppositional defiant disorder. Differences were less striking for attention-deficit/hyperactivity disorder, social phobia, agoraphobia, and substance abuse disorders. Ideation was more likely to be associated with adolescence and with a disruptive behavior disorder in younger children. The often-reported relation between panic disorder and suicide (J. Johnson et al. 1990; Weissman et al. 1989) is not sustained when comorbid depression is taken into account (Warshaw et al. 2000).

In addition to its relation to psychopathology, suicidal ideation is common in both the bullied and bullies (Kaltiala-Heino et al. 1999; Rigby and Slee 1999). It is significantly more common in gay, lesbian, and bisexual teenagers than in heterosexual teenagers (Blake et al. 2001; Faulkner and Cranston 1998; Fergusson et al. 1999; Garofalo et al. 1998; Lock and Steiner 1999; Remafedi et al. 1998). Gay, lesbian, and bisexual teenagers are more likely to be victimized at school (Garafalo et al. 1998), but it is not clear whether the relation between sexual orientation and suicidality is a direct consequence of their victimization or because gay, lesbian, and bisexual youths also have higher rates of drug and alcohol use and other psychiatric symptoms, such as major depression, generalized anxiety disorder, and conduct disorder (Fergusson et al. 1999).

Suicide Attempts

Definition and Subtypes

A suicide attempt is a common psychiatric symptom that occurs in children and teenagers with a variety of diagnoses and, less commonly, with no psychiatric disorders at all. Various attempts have been made to define meaningful subgroups among suicide attempters. The World Health Organization has defined a suicide attempt as

> an act with non-fatal outcome, in which an individual deliberately initiates a non-habitual behavior that, without intervention from others, will cause self-harm, or deliberately ingests a substance in excess of the prescribed or generally recognized therapeutic dosage, and which is aimed at realizing changes which the subject desired via the actual or expected physical consequences. (Platt et al. 1992, p. 99)

The World Health Organization definition omits any mention of a wish to *die* or the use of the broader concept of "self-harm" and thus reflects the reluctance of many to accept that all attempts are accompanied by lethal intent.

This definition owes something to Kreitman (1969), who coined the term *parasuicide*, which was used to describe ingestions or skin cutting, most often in girls and usually with a benign outcome. This is a familiar profile: most clinically referred attempts are in girls, most are by ingestion or cutting (see Lewinsohn et al. 1996), and nearly all attempts have a nonlethal outcome. In other words, the term *parasuicide* adds little value to the less-inferential term *attempted suicide*. The term *parasuicide* would be useful only if it defined a clinically or prognostically distinct subgroup.

The term *suicide gesture* implies that the suicidal behavior is conducted without lethal intent, as a "cry for help" or "to attract attention." The term lends itself to derogatory usage, with the inference that the behavior is manipulative and is a waste of the clinician's and family's time. Even though many teenagers take no action to prevent being discovered (Piacentini et al. 1991) or use methods that are unlikely to result in death (Harris and Myers 1997; Hawton et al. 1982a; Myers 1992; Piacentini et al. 1991), about half of the teenagers seen in an emergency department after an "attempt" say that at the time of their action, they wanted to die. Given these limitations, these terms are best avoided.

Finally, the Centers for Disease Control and Prevention (2000) classifies suicide attempts according to whether they elicited *medical attention*. This gives a good indication of service burden, but it may be a better indicator of method than intent. Medical attention is always influenced by ease of access, and the presence of an ingestant is more likely to prompt a search for medical interventions than a failed hanging, which might require no medical attention yet indicate greater psychiatric disturbance.

Precipitants

Suicide attempts, like completed suicides, usually follow some recent event that induced stress in the victim, commonly legal difficulties (Stanley and Barter 1970), actual or anticipated academic failure or punishment (Beautrais et al. 1997; Lewinsohn et al. 1996), a disrupted relationship, or a humiliation such as being bullied. The stress events or the way they are perceived and exaggerated may be the result of a teenager's underlying psychiatric disorder. The minority of attempters in whom no circumscribed precipitant (Hawton et al. 1982b; Kienhorst et al. 1995) can be identified should be evaluated carefully to rule out an underlying depression.

Psychiatric Disorder

Most teenaged attempters have a recent history of psychiatric illness (Andrews and Lewinsohn 1992; Beautrais et al. 1998; Fergusson and Lynskey 1995; Garrison et al. 1991b; Gould et al. 1998; Velez and

Cohen 1988), most commonly a mood disorder, often associated with a conduct, an anxiety, or a substance abuse disorder or, less often, an eating disorder. Suicide attempts also are associated with recurring episodes of aggressive, angry, and impulsive behavior (Gispert et al. 1985, 1987; Hawton et al. 1999; Kingsbury et al. 1999; Stein et al. 1998). Some evidence shows that the tendency to aggressive behavior is quite stable. Aggressive 8-year-olds are more than twice as likely as nonaggressive 8-year-olds to think about or attempt suicide at age 16 (Sourander et al. 2001).

As with ideators, in approximately a quarter of attempters, there is no evidence of sustained psychopathology (Gould et al. 1998).

Cognitive Style

Feelings of hopelessness are common among suicide attempters (Kienhorst et al. 1992; Morano et al. 1993; Steer et al. 1993; for negative studies, see Asarnow et al. 1987; Rotheram-Borus et al. 1990). However, in one study (Spirito et al. 1991), teenaged attempters were more likely to make *positive* or *grandiose attributions* than were psychiatric control subjects.

Family Factors

Many of the features of family life seen among suicide attempters also are seen in adolescents with nonsuicidal psychiatric disorders, such as a higher proportion living in a single-parent home (Groholt et al. 2000; Wichstrum 2000), high rates of parental psychiatric illness, marital and parent-child conflict (Asarnow 1992; Taylor and Stansfeld 1984; Trautman and Shaffer 1984), low levels of parental monitoring (R.A. King et al. 2001), and disputes over limit setting. Adolescent suicide attempters are more likely than healthy, but not depressed, control subjects to have been sexually and/or physically abused at some time in their lives (Brand et al. 1996; Swanston et al. 1999).

Completed Suicide

Method

In the United States, most teenagers commit suicide with firearms, usually legally owned, but often inadequately secured, rifles or shotguns. Only 20% of the firearm suicides in the United States are committed with handguns (National Center for Health Statistics 2000). Method varies greatly in different countries and communities and appears to be determined by some mix of customs and availability (Amos et al. 2001; Moens et al. 1988). In some countries, the supply of rapidly lethal ingestants, such as barbiturates, is restricted. In the United Kingdom, new packaging and retailing regulations for acetaminophen have reduced deaths and liver transplants caused by such overdoses. In countries with especially high female suicide rates (e.g., India and China), certain types of rapidly lethal ingestants are common (e.g., paraquat and organophosphate) (Eddleston et al. 1998; Haynes 1987; Jeyaratnam 1990). However, it is not clear that this is entirely a method effect, because a high female attempt rate is found in Asian communities in other countries (Bhugra et al. 1999).

Precipitants

Most adolescent suicides, like attempts, appear to be impulsive and are preceded by a stress event (Brent et al. 1993; Gould et al. 1996). Most commonly, these events are disciplinary crises, such as getting into trouble at school or with a law enforcement agency. Other common precipitants include a ruptured relationship with a boyfriend or girlfriend or a fight among friends (Brent et al. 1993; Gould et al. 1996).

Previous Attempts

Between 25% and 50% of the persons who commit suicide have made a previous known suicide attempt (Groholt et al. 1997). Previous attempts are more common in girls and among patients with a mood disorder at the time of their death (Shaffer et al. 1996).

Psychopathology

In most cases, research on the psychopathology of suicide comes from interviews with significant contacts of the deceased in a psychological autopsy study. Such studies consistently find that the large majority of suicides occur in teenagers with a psychiatric disturbance (Apter et al. 1993; Brent et al. 1999; Groholt et al. 1997; Ho et al. 1995; Marttunen et al. 1991, 1995; Shaffer et al. 1988, 1996). The most common forms of psychiatric disorder are

- *Some form of mood disorder,* which is found in about two-thirds of all suicides (Apter et al. 1993; Brent et al. 1999; Shaffer et al. 1988, 1996). In girls, this usually takes the form of an uncomplicated major depression, whereas in boys, it is often comorbid with conduct disorder and/or substance abuse (Shaffer et al. 1996).
- *Substance or alcohol abuse,* which is present in up to two-thirds of older boys (Brent et al. 1999; Shaffer et al. 1996) and usually is complicated by comorbid mood and/or conduct problems.
- An *anxiety disorder,* which is present in between a quarter and a third of all suicides (Brent et al. 1999; Shaffer et al. 1996), nearly always with an associated mood disorder. Performance and anticipatory anxiety are particularly prominent and are sometimes viewed by others as a sign of "perfectionism."
- *Conduct or oppositional defiant disorder,* which is present in between a third and a half of all suicides (Brent et al. 1999; Shaffer et al. 1996), more often among males and older teenagers and, again, often comorbid with a mood or substance abuse disorder.
- *Schizophrenia,* which is present in fewer than 10% of suicides in the child and adolescent age group. Thus, even though the suicide rate is greatly increased in schizophrenia, because of its rarity, it accounts for very few suicides.

Similar diagnoses are found among both boys and girls (Brent et al. 1999; Shaffer et al. 1996), but they differ markedly in their relative importance (Shaffer et al. 1996). In girls, the most significant risk factor for suicide is major depression, which increases the risk of suicide 20-fold (Shaffer et al. 1996). In boys, the most significant risk factor is a previous suicide attempt, which increases the risk more than 30-fold (Brent et al. 1999; Shaffer et al. 1996). Although alcohol abuse and disruptive behavior disorders are among the most prevalent diagnoses in suicide victims, their base rate in the general population is high, and their specific predictive value is, therefore, low.

Underlying Etiological Risk Factors

Biology

Perinatal Morbidity

Perinatal adversity, such as low birth weight and maternal alcohol use and smoking, is recorded more often in the birth records of teenagers who commit suicide (Jacobson et al. 1987; Salk et al. 1985) than in those of control subjects, even after controlling for premature death. It is not known whether the mechanisms of this relation are a direct consequence of a neuropathological entity or of some common maternal factor that predisposes to perinatal morbidity, later psychiatric illness, and so forth.

Family History

Teenagers who complete suicide are between two and four times more likely than matched control subjects to have a first-degree relative who committed suicide (Brent et al. 1996; Shaffer et al. 1996). This is similar to the findings among adults who commit suicide (for a review, see Roy et al. 2000). A similar relation has been reported in a community-based study of suicide attempters (Bridge et al. 1997; B. A. Johnson et al. 1998).

A family history of suicidal behavior is an independent risk factor after accounting for parent psychiatric diagnoses (Brent et al. 1996; Gould et al. 1996). Both adopted-away (Schulsinger et al. 1979) and twin studies (Roy et al. 2000; Statham et al. 1998) suggest that the relationship has a genetic basis and is not simply a consequence of being reared by a psychiatrically ill parent.

Serotonergic Abnormalities

In 1976, Åsberg et al. noted a relation between low levels of cerebrospinal fluid 5-hydroxyindoleacetic acid (5-HIAA), the major metabolite of serotonin, and a prior suicide attempt in a group of adult patients with melancholic depression. This has now become one of the most replicated findings in biological psychiatry (for a review, see Oquendo and Mann 2000). Autoradiographic studies suggest that the abnormality is presynaptic and results in compensatory upregulation of postsynaptic serotonin type 2 receptors in the ventral and ventrolateral prefrontal cortex—the area of the central nervous system that is in large measure responsible for behavioral inhibition. If this is confirmed, it also might explain the relation between serotonergic dysfunction and aggressivity.

Mann et al. (1999) proposed a stress-diathesis model. In this model, they proposed that dysregulation is a biological trait. A mentally ill individual who has this trait is more likely to respond to a stressful experience in an impulsive and aggressive fashion, starting and maintaining a vicious cycle of stress that leads to inappropriate responses, which in turn generate more stress. The decision to commit suicide is seen as the ultimate intense and ill-considered response (see Figure 5–3).

These findings have led to an active investigation of two candidate genes: the promoter region of the serotonin transporter gene and the gene for tryptophan hydroxylase, the rate-limiting enzyme for the synthesis of serotonin. Research findings on these candidate genes have been inconsistent (Bennett et al. 2000; Geijer et al. 2000; Nielsen et al. 1994, 1998; Ohara et al. 1998; Rujescu et al. 2001). It is not clear whether this is because the suicide phenotype comprises many different etiological factors, because the genetic effect is small and requires the analysis of many patients, or because the clinical importance of a single genetic variant might not be apparent unless studied with other related genes (Marshall et al. 1999).

Despite the numerous studies that have reported these abnormalities, some unanswered questions remain. The specific behavioral correlates of low serotonin states have yet to be documented in representative samples of suicide completers, conflicting reports exist about whether 5-HIAA levels are stable or fluctuate with mental state, and the proportion of teenaged or adult suicide victims with such abnormalities has yet to be determined.

The biological findings should eventually influence clinical

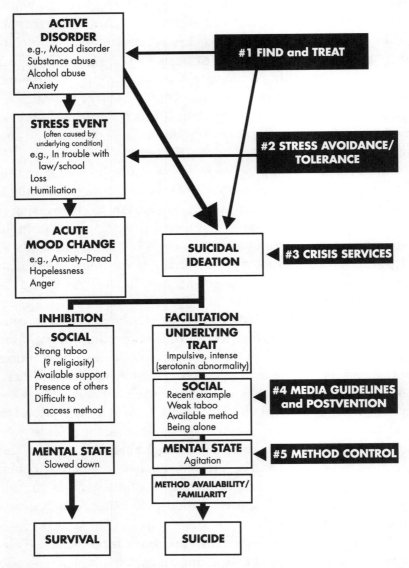

Figure 5–3. How do suicides occur and how can they be prevented?

practice. Nordstrom et al. (1994) found that suicide attempters with low levels of cerebrospinal fluid 5-HIAA were significantly more likely to make a future attempt and/or to commit suicide. If declining or stable low levels of 5-HIAA predict a poor prognosis, then secondary or tertiary prevention could be served by routine cerebrospinal fluid monitoring of the patients who have attempted suicide, with special care being given to those with abnormally low levels.

Imitation and Contagion

Evidence shows that, at least in the young with prior psychiatric problems, both attempted and completed suicide can be provoked by exposure to presentations of suicide-related material in the media (for a review, see Velting and Gould 1997). The evidence includes single case accounts of teenagers who committed suicide shortly after seeing a film or television program or reading a book or news story about a suicide (Shaffer 1974) and the occurrence of well-documented clusters of suicide within a given geographical area within a limited time. Cluster suicides are estimated to account for up to 4% of all teenage suicides in the United States (Gould 1990).

Several studies showed a relation in time between the occurrence of a published or broadcast account of a suicide and a subsequent increase in suicide and suicide attempt rates among those who were likely to have been exposed to the account (Gould and Shaffer 1986; Gould et al. 1988; Holding 1974, 1975; Schmidtke and Hafner 1986; Sonneck et al. 1994). The excess of suicides that follow such a broadcast or publication lasts between 7 and 14 days and is related to the number of times that the news story is repeated (Bollen and Phillips 1981, 1982; Phillips 1974, 1979, 1980, 1984; Wasserman 1984). The effect of a single stimulus is likely to vary with the age and size of the exposed viewership and the context in which the material is seen (e.g., whether the programs were accompanied by material that could direct a disturbed viewer to obtain help). This has been the case with individual programs (Berman 1988; Gould et al. 1988). They are generally termed *ecological* because they do not establish whether a given person who committed suicide was or was not exposed to the stimulus. In the most convincing of these studies, Schmidtke and Hafner (1986) reported on the broadcast of a fictional television program that featured a 19-year-old boy's suicide on a railway track. This was followed by a sharp, but time-limited, increase in suicides using the same method. When the series was rebroadcast 1 year later, the same phenomenon occurred.

Little is known about the mechanism of contagion in adult populations. Philips (1984) found that the effect of news stories was primarily on the very young, and some evidence indicates that older populations have a different response. In a study conducted between 1992 and 1995, Mercy and colleagues (2001) compared a series of 153 predominantly adult, near-lethal suicide attempters seen in an emergency department with community control subjects. The group failed to find a relation between making a serious suicide attempt and exposure to the suicidal behavior of a relative or accounts of suicide in the media. More than three quarters of the sample was adult, and the high-school-age subpopulation comprised about 30 subjects. In that study, the predominantly adult attempters were less likely to know of a suicidal friend or acquaintance.

Family Circumstances

In one case-controlled study (Gould et al. 1996) that compared adolescents who committed suicide with nonsuicidal control subjects, adolescents who committed suicide were less likely than nonsuicidal control subjects to live with both of their biological parents. But parent-child discord was not a risk factor, and discord between parents and parental divorce increased risk only slightly, although suicidal adolescents were significantly more likely to have infrequent or dissatisfactory communications with their parents.

Drug-Induced Suicidality

In the past decade, whether SSRI antidepressants can induce suicidal ideation and/or behavior in both adults (Teicher et al. 1990) and children (R. A. King et al. 1991) has been controversial. This was supported by one meta-analysis (Mann and Kapur 1991), and a few adult cases have been reported in which suicidal thoughts started after treatment was begun with an SSRI, stopped after its withdrawal, and reappeared once the drug was recommenced (Rothschild and Locke 1991). Many of the case reports showed that the ideation was associated with akathisia and that it had an obsessive or a ruminative quality (Hamilton and Opler 1992). These suicidogenic effects of the SSRIs are probably uncommon, and meta-analyses and reanalyses of large sets of SSRI-treatment-trial data of depressed, bulimic, or anxious patients (Beasley et al. 1991; Letizia et al. 1996; Montgomery et al. 1995) suggest that the overall effect is for the medication to reduce rates of suicidal behavior. Nevertheless, clinicians should be particularly observant during the early stages of SSRI treatment, should systematically inquire about suicidal ideation before and after treatment is started, and should, if SSRI treatment induces akathisia, be especially alert to the possibility of suicidality.

Assessment and Treatment

Suicidal Ideation

Suicidal ideation is rarely chosen as a dependent variable in treatment research, and the references here are probably incomplete. In general, the management of suicidal ideation involves the management of any associated disorders. However, given the key role of ideation in determining attempts and completions, it would seem to be a legitimate target for treatment. SSRI antidepressants have been shown to reduce suicidal ideation in both depressed (Letizia et al. 1996) and nondepressed patients with Cluster B personality disorders (Verkes et al. 1998b) and in individuals who have made a limited number of previous suicide attempts. SSRIs are, in general, safe and effective for adolescent depression (Emslie et al. 1997; Ryan and Varma 1998) and are significantly less dangerous in overdose than are tricyclic antidepressants (Ryan and Varma 1998). Pending evidence to the contrary, it would be reasonable to regard SSRIs as a first-choice medication for depressed, suicidal adolescents.

In rare instances, ruminative suicidal ideation combined with akathisia can be induced by an antipsychotic or by an SSRI. This complication has been reported to respond to propranolol (Adler et al. 1985; Chandler 1990).

Cognitive-behavioral therapy reduced suicidal ideation in a sample of college students (Lerner and Clum 1990).

Suicide Attempts and Completed Suicide

Emergency Care

Suicide attempters are commonly seen in an emergency department; after medical stabilization, a decision must be made about whether they need admission. Admission is unambiguously indicated for those with an abnormal mental state, especially if characterized by agitation or irritability, and for the small proportion of attempters who state that they have a persistent wish to die. Clinical features that are associated with suicide attempts or later suicide are listed in Table 5–2, and the decision to admit a patient is often made by an imprecise juggling of these risks. The risk of suicide is remote in children aged 12 or younger, and suicidal ideation or behavior should not, by themselves, be an indication for hospitalization in that age group. Until we know more about the positive or negative effect of hospitalization (C. A. King et al. 1995; Waterhouse and Platt 1990), decisions on whether to admit a recent attempter who is euthymic often will be based on essentially nonclinical considerations, such as insurance coverage and bed availability. Many admissions are perforce brief and are made to hospitals that are organizationally and geographically distinct and might have quite different staff from where the patient will receive follow-up care. Whether these seemingly negative features of inpatient care affect outcome is simply not known.

The parent who accompanies the patient to the emergency department should be told, before discharge, to limit the adolescent's access to alcohol or other potentially disinhibiting substances and to lock away poisonous medications and firearms. Parents accept and comply with these instructions when given clearly (Kruesi et al. 1999), and in their absence parents might do little to make firearms more secure (Brent et al. 2000).

"Contracts for safety" are commonly drawn up between the patient and the clinician before discharge. These require the patient to contact the clinician first before making any further attempt. However, the effect of these contracts has never been

Table 5–2.   Factors to consider when deciding whether to hospitalize an adolescent

Strong indicators for hospitalization

Markedly abnormal mental state

Persistent wish to die

Highly lethal or unusual method

Factors that favor hospitalization but that are not in themselves sufficient

Prior attempt(s)

Male sex

Family history of suicide

Inadequate care and supervision at home

Aged 16 years or older

Contraindications to hospitalization

No Factor I categories *and:* prepubertal *or* only small overdose or superficial cutting

---

assessed, and facilitating access between patient and clinician has not been shown to alter the reattempt rate (Cotgrove et al. 1995). It would be sensible to assume that risk can persist even if the patient has contracted for safety (Drew 2001; Egan et al. 1997; Reid 1998).

Long-Term Psychopharmacological Treatment

In adults with bipolar or other major mood disorders, long-term lithium treatment significantly reduces the recurrence of suicide attempts (Tondo et al. 1997). The antisuicidal effects of lithium have not been assessed in children or adolescents.

In a controlled trial of the depot neuroleptic flupenthixol, Montgomery et al. (1979) noted a significant reduction in suicide attempt behavior in adults who had made numerous previous attempts. This study has not been replicated, and similar studies have not been done with adolescents.

Psychotherapy

The only form of psychotherapy that has been shown in a randomized clinical trial to reduce multiple attempts is dialectical behavior therapy (DBT) (Linehan et al. 1991, 1994) (see below). Treatments that have failed to yield an improvement include problem-solving therapies with standard care (see Hawton et al. 1998, 2000b), enhanced access to a clinical service (Cotgrove et al. 1995; Hawton et al. 1981, 2000b; Rotheram-Borus et al. 2000; van der Sande et al. 1997), and home-based family therapy (Harrington et al. 1998).

DBT was developed by Linehan et al. (1991, 1993) for adult suicide attempters to address the problems of poor emotional regulation that are commonly found in attempters.

As described, DBT is given in several sessions a week for approximately a year. Its components include 1) training in self-acceptance, 2) increasing assertiveness to reduce interpersonal conflicts, 3) training the patient to avoid situations that trigger negative moods, and 4) increasing tolerance of distress. DBT-A is an adaptation developed for adolescents (A. L. Miller et al. 1997). It is given for 6 months, rather than a year, but has not yet been tested in a controlled study.

No studies of cognitive-behavioral therapy in the suicidal teenager have been recorded, although it has been used successfully in teenaged patients with depression (Birmaher et al. 2000; Harrington and Clark 1998).

In the absence of evidence for a "best" therapy, the clinician may sensibly choose to 1) treat any associated psychiatric disorder, 2) teach the patient and the family to recognize and then avoid or diffuse situations that could lead to conflict or distress (S. Miller et al. 1992), and 3) improve the morale and sense of capability that are commonly damaged in the families of teenagers who have attempted suicide (K. E. Miller et al. 1992; Stuart 1980; Trautman and Shaffer 1984).

Compliance

Slightly fewer than half of the suicide attempters who present in crisis eventually will develop a therapeutic relationship after their initial evaluation and treatment (Kienhorst et al. 1987; Litt et al. 1983; Piacentini et al. 1991; Spirito et al. 1989; Swedo 1989; Taylor and Stansfield 1984; Trautman and Rotheram-Borus 1988). If a suicide attempter does not return to the clinic, the reason is unlikely to be that he or she is "doing well." Trautman and Shaffer (1989) and Piacentini et al. (1991) found that nonattendance was more common in attempters who were persistently suicidal, in those who had many psychiatric symptoms, and, less consistently, in those whose mothers abused drugs or alcohol or were in poor physical health.

Prevention

A complicated chain of events and moods (see Figure 5–3) likely leads to the moment when a teenager decides to commit suicide. An examination of this pathway suggests a number of points for intervention.

Underlying Disorder

Nearly all patients who commit suicide have a mental illness at the time of their death, usually a mood disorder, although a history of attempted suicide, current ideation, and substance abuse increases the risk. Finding individual patients with those characteristics is the cornerstone of prevention. The two most commonly used techniques for case finding are 1) direct screening combined with case management to treatment and 2) educating third parties to identify the characteristics of a suicidal teenager and persuade them to seek treatment.

Screening

Direct screening can be done in pediatric and adolescent health clinics or in locations where high-risk teenagers congregate (e.g., school guidance offices, juvenile justice facilities, and shelters for runaway youths). Indirect screening can be done by administering surveys to adult psychiatric patients who have a greatly increased likelihood of having a teenaged child with a mood disorder.

Systematic screening usually entails use of a brief self-report measure to assess current suicidal ideation, a history of suicide attempts, depressed mood, and substance abuse (Goldston 2000; Harkavy-Friedman et al. 1987; Shaffer and Craft 1999; Smith and

Crawford 1986). Some measures focus narrowly on suicidality (Beck et al. 1979; Pfeffer et al. 2000; Reynolds 1987; Tatman et al. 1993), but these may not include risk factors, such as depression and substance abuse, that can set the stage for future suicidality. Self-report measures can be extremely sensitive, correlate well with the findings of clinicians (Renouf and Kovacs 1994), and, indeed, often identify teenagers who were not selected by teachers or parents (Achenbach and Edelbrock 1987; Bird et al. 1990; Kovacs 1985). Broad or generic self-completion instruments, such as the Youth Self-Report (Achenbach and Edelbrock 1987), that incorporate a very wide range of symptoms likely have poor specificity for suicide risk and thus produce a high false-positive rate. Focused screening instruments, such as the Columbia Teen-Screen, are very sensitive (i.e., have the potential for identifying most suicidal teenagers) but identify many false-positive results. This means that unless students who have a positive screen can be given a second-stage evaluation, a single screen likely will create an unmanageable service burden (Reynolds 1991; Shaffer and Craft 1999). In a screen of more than 2,000 New York teenagers (Shaffer and Craft 1999), the initial screen generated only 3 false-negative results (88% sensitivity) but 257 false-positive results (70% specificity). Adding a second-stage procedure—in this case, the Diagnostic Interview Schedule for Children, Version IV, a low-cost, self-administered, computerized diagnostic interview (Shaffer et al. 2000)—reduced the proportion of students who had to be seen by a clinician by 60% but only marginally reduced the number of students who would go on to experience a later suicide attempt or depression.

Education Programs for Teenagers, Parents, and Teachers

An alternative approach to case finding is to educate parents, teachers, and guidance personnel about suggestive behavior patterns or warning signs. Such a "universalist" strategy will present the educational program to mostly teenagers or families who have no risk for suicide, and if directed to teenagers, it can be problematic. It requires presenting material about suicide to groups of teenagers, and this creates the risk of perturbing unidentified formerly or currently suicidal students (Shaffer et al. 1991). Most programs require a teenager to either persuade a friend who has shown depression or suicidality to obtain help themselves or, if that fails, disclose their observations to a responsible adult. These are daunting tasks for a teenager, and it should be no surprise that students who have received systematic training in counseling their friends to obtain help are no more likely to do so than are control subjects who received no training (Shaffer et al. 1990, 1991; Spirito et al. 1988; Vieland et al. 1991).

Professional Education for Physicians

Even though primary care physicians commonly prescribe antidepressants to adolescent patients (Goodwin et al. 2001; Rushton and Whitmire 2001), considerably fewer than half of physicians and pediatricians regularly ask their patients about suicide risk conditions (Frankenfield et al. 2000; Halpern-Felsher et al. 2000). Professional education to primary care physicians to teach them how to best identify and treat suicidality in teenaged patients can be helpful in this regard. This was shown on the Swedish island of Gotland (Rihmer et al. 1995; Rutz et al. 1992), where a 2-day training program for primary care physicians on how to assess mood disorders and suicidality was associated with a significant reduction in the female suicide rate (Rihmer et al. 1995; Rutz et al. 1995) and an increase in antidepressant prescriptions and hospitalizations for mood disorders.

Stress Events

Stresses commonly precede a suicide or attempted suicide (Brent et al. 1993; Gould et al. 1996). For the most part, these are common teenage stresses and could not be reasonably eliminated. However, treatments such as DBT (Linehan et al. 1993) emphasize stress avoidance and stress tolerance in suicidal individuals and may be one of the reasons that treatment is effective. Attempts have been made to teach these skills prophylactically to unselected teenagers (Friedberg et al. 2001), but the clinical use of these approaches has a highly personal orientation, and it is difficult to see how more generic "coping skills" classes could be of value to vulnerable high-risk teenagers. Psychopharmacological treatments may exert a preventive effect at this point, both by reducing the generation of new stresses and by lowering the affective response to stresses when experienced.

Active Suicidal Ideation

Acute psychological distress nearly always precedes a suicidal event. Crisis services originally were set up to be helpful to individuals, many of whom are ambivalent about their wish to die (Shneidman and Farberow 1957).

Crisis services usually are provided by telephone or so-called hot lines. Some are staffed by teenagers (Boehm et al. 1991; Simmons et al. 1986), but most have specially trained adult helpers. Some provide active case management, making appointments with convenient clinical services and following up if the appointment is not kept (Sudak et al. 1977). A few offer confidential telephone therapy, such as the Samaritans' befriending technique that emphasizes acceptance and warmth (Hirsch 1981). Others will break confidentiality if they judge that doing so will avert a suicide.

No information exists on the extent to which highly suicidal individuals are redirected from their intended plan by contact with a crisis service. Most evaluations of crisis intervention have been tested ecologically by examining changes in the suicide rate in a population before and after the establishment of a crisis service. These rarely lowered suicide morbidity in the area under study (for a review, see Mishara and Daigle 2000). Factors that limit the potential for hot lines to reduce the suicide rate include

- *Caller characteristics.* Most callers are female (Boehm and Campbell 1995), who, even after a suicide attempt, are at low risk for suicide. A high proportion of callers are not suicidal, whereas many suicidal teenagers, despite knowledge of hot lines, do not call (Offer et al. 1991; Vieland et al. 1991).
- *Helper characteristics.* Helpers have a high turnover rate and often are not trained to give advice or help specific to the circumstances or mental state of the caller (Hirsch 1981; Knowles 1979; Slaiku et al. 1975).

- *Methodological problems.* Even if crisis services were effective, their efficacy could not be confirmed unless the service collected information in order to do short- and long-term follow-up studies.

Social Provocation

An underlying disorder, recent stress, and the affective responses to stress set the stage for suicidal ideation. Given the high rate of ideation and of psychiatric symptoms among ideators, one expects that many teenagers reach this stage. But very few will go on to commit suicide. At this point, specific "enhancers" and "restrainers" probably operate.

Witnessing news or seeing a film can increase the risk for suicide. Preventive interventions operating at this penultimate stage could include media guidelines to promote responsible reporting of suicide to minimize the risk of contagion. The American Foundation for Suicide Prevention (2001) has prepared guidelines for minimizing the effect of reporting on an individual suicide, including placing the story in a less prominent position within print media, avoiding romanticizing or idealizing the suicide victim, and not providing details of the method that could allow modeling.

To date, only limited research has been done on the effectiveness of such guidelines (Etzersdorfer et al. 1992; Jobes et al. 1996; Sonneck et al. 1994).

School-based postventions are interventions implemented *after* a suicide with survivors in the victim's school or community. An integral concern of all postvention activities is to prevent imitation. Postvention programs also offer some understanding of the causes of death, thus reducing some of the scapegoating that might be directed to family, teachers, and peers (Calhoun et al. 1982; Henley 1984; Rogers et al. 1982). It is not clear how postvention programs might reduce the probability of imitation by other teenagers. The only controlled study on postvention (Hazell and Lewin 1993) found no significant improvement in symptoms of the students who were close friends of the teenager who committed suicide and who attended postvention group sessions.

However, because most participants in a suicide cluster were symptomatic before their death (Gould 2001), one approach might be to screen survivors for high-risk status and then direct individual attention to them.

Method Access

Because youth suicide is often an impulsive act, it is reasonable to expect that limiting access to commonly used methods could prevent its occurrence in certain instances. The so-called British experience, when natural gas replaced coal gas, is a frequently cited example of the striking but transient effect of reducing the availability of a commonly used method. A second, more recent British experience has been the effect of limiting the packaging size of acetaminophen, on the assumption that this will reduce the impulsive ingestion of potentially lethal quantities of that medication. This appears to have resulted in a significant reduction in suicidal deaths attributable to acetaminophen and also to a striking reduction in liver transplants performed on survivors of toxic ingestions (Hawton et al. 2001, in press).

Most suicides in the United States are committed with legally owned and registered firearms. One might expect that the early British experience could be replicated by effective firearm control, but, by extension, one would expect a similarly transient effect.

Because it is impossible to restrict access to common methods such as hanging and jumping, one can only agree with Beautrais (2000) that method restriction is a generally flawed approach to suicide prevention.

Conclusion

If the suicide rate continues its striking decline, we can hope that death from depression will be a condition of the past. It seems likely that the decline is a product of more widely administered and more effective treatment. This means that the burden on professionals to identify depressed and suicidal teenagers and bring them to treatment is greater than ever before.

Given the burden of suicidality, there is a great need for more information on optimal treatment. The quality of psychopharmacological research on suicidality is generally poor; most studies are small and unreplicated. This is especially unfortunate because of the efficacy of psychotropic medication in other conditions, its low cost, and its transportability. Well-designed studies on candidate medications must be conducted as a matter of urgency. DBT, the only form of psychotherapy that has been shown to be effective in adult attempters, needs to be studied in young people, along with ways to reduce its cost and complexity.

References

Achenbach TM, Edelbrock C: Manual for the Youth Self-Report and Profile. Burlington, University of Vermont, Department of Psychiatry, 1987

Adler L, Angrist B, Peselow E, et al: Efficacy of propranolol in neuroleptic-induced akathesia. J Clin Psychopharmacol 5:164–166, 1985

American Foundation for Suicide Prevention, Gould MS, Kramer R: Reporting a suicide. 2001. Available at: http://www.afsp.org

Amos T, Appleby L, Kiernan K: Changes in rates of suicide by car-exhaust asphyxiation in England and Wales. Psychol Med 31:935–939, 2001

Andersen UA, Andersen M, Rosholm JU, et al: Psychopharmacological treatment and psychiatric morbidity in 390 cases of suicide with special focus on affective disorders. Acta Psychiatr Scand 104:458–465, 2001

Andrews JA, Lewinsohn PM: Suicidal attempts among older adolescents: prevalence and co-occurrence with psychiatric disorders. J Am Acad Child Adolesc Psychiatry 31:655–662, 1992

Apter A, Bleich A, King RA, et al: Death without warning? A clinical postmortem study of suicide in 43 Israeli adolescent males. Arch Gen Psychiatry 50:138–142, 1993

Asarnow JR: Suicidal ideation and attempts during middle childhood: associations with perceived family stress and depression among child psychiatric inpatients. J Clin Child Psychol 21:35–40, 1992

Asarnow JR, Carlson GA, Guthrie D: Coping strategies, self-perceptions, hopelessness, and perceived family environments in depressed and suicidal children. J Consult Clin Psychol 55:361–366, 1987

Åsberg M, Thorén P, Träskman L, et al: "Serotonin depression"—a biochemical subgroup within the affective disorders? Science 191:478–480, 1976

Australian Bureau of Statistics: Mortality data. Injury deaths for 1988–2000, supplied upon written request to the National Information and Referral Service at client.services@abs.gov.au. Contacted December 6, 2001

Beasley CMJ, Dornseif BE, Bosomworth JC, et al: Fluoxetine and suicide: a meta-analysis of controlled trials of treatment for depression. BMJ 303:685–692, 1991

Beautrais AL: Methods of youth suicide in New Zealand: trends and implications for prevention. Aust N Z J Psychiatry 34:413–419, 2000

Beautrais AL, Joyce PR, Mulder RT: Precipitating factors and life events in serious suicide attempts among youths aged 13 through 24 years. J Am Acad Child Adolesc Psychiatry 36:1543–1551, 1997

Beautrais AL, Joyce PR, Mulder RT: Psychiatric illness in a New Zealand sample of young people making serious suicide attempts. N Z Med J 111:44–48, 1998

Beck AT, Kovacs M, Weissman A: Assessment of suicidal intention: the Scale for Suicide Ideation. J Consult Clin Psychol 47:343–352, 1979

Bennett PJ, McMahon WM, Watabe J, et al: Tryptophan hydroxylase polymorphisms in suicide victims. Psychiatr Genet 10:13–17, 2000

Berman AL: Fictional depiction of suicide in television films and imitation effects. Am J Psychiatry 145:982–986, 1988

Bhugra D, Desai M, Baldwin DS: Attempted suicide in West London, I: rates across ethnic communities. Psychol Med 29:1125–1130, 1999

Bird HR, Yager TJ, Staghezza B, et al: Impairment in the epidemiological measurement of childhood psychopathology in the community. J Am Acad Child Adolesc Psychiatry 29:796–803, 1990

Birmaher B, Brent DA, Kolko D, et al: Clinical outcome after short-term psychotherapy for adolescents with major depressive disorder. Arch Gen Psychiatry 57:29–36, 2000

Blake SM, Ledsky R, Lehman T, et al: Preventing sexual risk behaviors among gay, lesbian, and bisexual adolescents: the benefits of gay-sensitive HIV instruction in schools. Am J Public Health 91:940–946, 2001

Boehm K, Chessare JB, Valko TR, et al: Teen Line: a descriptive analysis of a peer telephone listening service. Adolescence 26:643–648, 1991

Boehm KE, Campbell NB: Suicide: a review of calls to an adolescent peer listening phone service. Child Psychiatry Hum Dev 26:61–66, 1995

Bollen KA, Phillips DP: Suicidal motor vehicle fatalities in Detroit: a replication. American Journal of Sociology 87:404–412, 1981

Bollen KA, Philips DP: Imitative suicides: a national study of the effects of television news stories. Am Sociol Rev 47:802–809, 1982

Brand EF, King CA, Olson E, et al: Depressed adolescents with a history of sexual abuse: diagnostic comorbidity and suicidality. J Am Acad Child Adolesc Psychiatry 5:34–41, 1996

Brent DA, Perper JA, Moritz G, et al: Psychiatric risk factors for adolescent suicide: a case-control study. J Am Acad Child Adolesc Psychiatry 32:521–529, 1993

Brent DA, Bridge J, Johnson BA, et al: Suicidal behavior runs in families: a controlled family study of adolescent suicide victims. Arch Gen Psychiatry 53:1145–1152, 1996

Brent DA, Baugher M, Bridge J, et al: Age- and sex-related risk factors for adolescent suicide. J Am Acad Child Adolesc Psychiatry 38:1497–1505, 1999

Brent DA, Baugher M, Birmaher B, et al: Compliance with recommendations to remove firearms in families participating in a clinical trial for adolescent depression. J Am Acad Child Adolesc Psychiatry 39:1220–1226, 2000

Bridge JA, Brent D, Johnson BA, et al: Familial aggregation of psychiatric disorders in a community sample of adolescents. J Am Acad Child Adolesc Psychiatry 36:628–636, 1997

Bush JA: Suicide and blacks: a conceptual framework. Suicide Life Threat Behav 6:216–222, 1976

Calhoun LG, Selby JW, Selby LE: The psychological aftermath of suicide: an analysis of current evidence. Clin Psychol Rev 2:409–420, 1982

Centers for Disease Control and Prevention: Youth Risk Behavior Surveillance National Alternative High-School Youth Risk Behavior Survey, United States, 1998. MMWR Morb Mortal Wkly Rep 48 (No. 55–57):12, 1999

Centers for Disease Control and Prevention: Youth Risk Behavior Surveillance—United States, 1999. MMWR Morb Mortal Wkly Rep 49:1–95, 2000

Central Statistics Office Ireland: Injury deaths Ireland 1988–2000, supplied upon written request to http://www.cso.ie. Contacted September 5, 2001

Chandler JD: Propranolol treatment of akathisia in Tourette's syndrome. J Am Acad Child Adolesc Psychiatry 29:475–477, 1990

Cheng AT: Mental illness and suicide: a case-control study in east Taiwan. Arch Gen Psychiatry 52:594–603, 1995

Chew KS, McCleary R: The spring peak in suicides: a cross-national analysis. Soc Sci Med 40:223–230, 1995

Choquet M, Menke H: Suicidal thoughts during early adolescence: prevalence, associated troubles and help-seeking behavior. Acta Psychiatr Scand 81:170–177, 1989

Chung SY, Luk SL, Mak FL: Attempted suicide in children and adolescents in Hong Kong. Soc Psychiatry 22:102–106, 1987

Cotgrove A, Zirinsky L, Black D, et al: Secondary prevention of attempted suicide in adolescence. J Adolesc 18:569–577, 1995

Drew BL: Self-harm behavior and no-suicide contracting in psychiatric inpatient settings. Arch Psychiatr Nurs 15:99–106, 2001

Dubow EF: Correlates of suicidal ideation and attempts in a community sample of junior and high-school students. J Clin Child Psychol 18:158–166, 1989

Eastwood MR, Peter AM: Epidemiology and seasonal affective disorder. Psychol Med 18:799–806, 1988

Eddleston M, Sheriff MH, Hawton K: Deliberate self-harm in Sri Lanka: an overlooked tragedy in the developing world. BMJ 317:133–135, 1998

Egan MP, Rivera SG, Robillard RR, et al: The "no suicide contract": helpful or harmful? J Psychosoc Nurs Ment Health Serv 35:31–33, 1997

Emslie GJ, Rush AJ, Weinberg WA, et al: A double-blind, randomized, placebo-controlled trial of fluoxetine in children and adolescents with depression. Arch Gen Psychiatry 54:1031–1037, 1997

Etzersdorfer E, Sonneck G, Nagel-Kuess S: Newspaper reports and suicide (letter). N Engl J Med 327:502–503, 1992

Faulkner AH, Cranston K: Correlates of same-sex sexual behavior in a random sample of Massachusetts high-school students. Am J Public Health 88:262–266, 1998

Fergusson DM, Lynskey MT: Suicide attempts and suicidal ideation in a birth cohort of 16-year-old New Zealanders. J Am Acad Child Adolesc Psychiatry 34:1308–1317, 1995

Fergusson DM, Horwood LJ, Beautrais AL: Is sexual orientation related to mental health problems and suicidality in young people? Arch Gen Psychiatry 56:876–880, 1999

Flisher AJ, Parry CD, Bradshaw D, et al: Seasonal variation of suicide in South Africa. Psychiatry Res 66:13–22, 1997

Frankenfield DL, Keyl PM, Gielen A, et al: Adolescent patients—healthy or hurting? Missed opportunities to screen for suicide risk in the primary care setting. Arch Pediatr Adolesc Med 154:162–168, 2000

Friedberg RD, Friedberg BA, Friedberg RJ: Therapeutic Exercises for Children: Guided Self-Discovery Using Cognitive-Behavioral Techniques. Sarasota, FL, Professional Resource Press/Professional Resource Exchange, 2001

Garofalo R, Wolf RC, Kessel S, et al: The association between health risk behaviors and sexual orientation among a school-based sample of adolescents. Pediatrics 101:895–902, 1998

Garrison CZ, Addy CL, Jackson KL, et al: A longitudinal study of suicidal ideation in young adolescents. J Am Acad Child Adolesc Psychiatry 30:597–603, 1991a

Garrison CZ, Jackson KL, Addy CL, et al: Suicidal behaviors in young adolescents. Am J Epidemiol 133:1005–1014, 1991b

Geijer T, Frisch A, Persson ML, et al: Search for association between suicide attempt and serotonergic polymorphisms. Psychiatr Genet 10: 19–26, 2000

Gibbs J, Martin W: Status Integration and Suicide. Eugene, University of Oregon Press, 1964

Gispert M, Wheeler K, Marsh L, et al: Suicidal adolescents: factors in evaluation. Adolescence 20:753–762, 1985

Gispert M, Davis MS, Marsh L, et al: Predictive factors in repeated suicide attempts by adolescents. Hospital and Community Psychiatry 38:390–393, 1987

Goldacre M, Hawton K: Repetition of self-poisoning and subsequent death in adolescents who take overdoses. Br J Psychiatry 146:395–398, 1985

Goldston DB: Assessment of suicidal behaviors and risk among children and adolescents. Technical report submitted to National Institute of Mental Health under contract 263-MD-909995. 2000. Available at: http://www.nimh.nih.gov/research/measures

Goodwin FK, Jamison KR: Manic-Depressive Illness. New York, Oxford University Press, 1990

Goodwin R, Gould MS, Blanco C, et al: Prescription of psychotropic medications to youths in office-based practice. Psychiatr Serv 52: 1081–1087, 2001

Gould MS: Suicide clusters and media exposure, in Suicide Over the Life Cycle: Risk Factors, Assessment, and Treatment of Suicidal Patients. Edited by Blumenthal SJ, Kupfer DJ. Washington, DC, American Psychiatric Press, 1990, pp 517–532

Gould MS: Suicide and the media, in The Clinical Science of Suicide Prevention. Edited by Hendin H, Mann JJ. New York, New York Academy of Sciences, 2001, pp 200–224

Gould MS, Shaffer D: The impact of suicide in television movies: evidence of imitation [published erratum appears in N Engl J Med 319: 1616, 1988]. N Engl J Med 315:690–694, 1986

Gould MS, Shaffer D, Kleinman M: The impact of suicide in television movies: replication and commentary. Suicide Life Threat Behav 18: 90–99, 1988

Gould MS, Fisher P, Parides M, et al: Psychosocial risk factors of child and adolescent completed suicide. Arch Gen Psychiatry 53:1155–1162, 1996

Gould MS, King R, Greenwald S, et al: Psychopathology associated with suicidal ideation and attempts among children and adolescents. J Am Acad Child Adolesc Psychiatry 37:915–923, 1998

Groholt B, Ekeberg O, Wichstrom L, et al: Youth suicide in Norway, 1990–1992: a comparison between children and adolescents completing suicide and age- and gender-matched controls. Suicide Life Threat Behav 27:250–263, 1997

Groholt B, Ekeberg O, Wichstrom L, et al: Young suicide attempters: a comparison between a clinical and an epidemiological sample. J Am Acad Child Adolesc Psychiatry 39:868–875, 2000

Hakko H, Rasanen P, Tiihonen J: Secular trends in the rates and seasonality of violent and nonviolent suicide occurrences in Finland during 1980–95. J Affect Disord 50:49–54, 1998

Halpern-Felsher BL, Ozer EM, Millstein SG, et al: Preventive services in a health maintenance organization: how well do pediatricians screen and educate adolescent patients? Arch Pediatr Adolesc Med 154: 173–179, 2000

Hamilton MS, Opler LA: Akathisia, suicidality, and fluoxetine. J Clin Psychiatry 53:401–406, 1992

Harkavy Friedman JM, Asnis GM, Boeck M, et al: Prevalence of specific suicidal behaviors in a high-school sample. Am J Psychiatry 144: 1203–1206, 1987

Harrington R, Clark A: Prevention and early intervention for depression in adolescence and early adult life. Eur Arch Psychiatry Clin Neurosci 248:32–45, 1998

Harrington R, Kerfoot M, Dyer E, et al: Randomized trial of a home-based family intervention for children who have deliberately poisoned themselves. J Am Acad Child Adolesc Psychiatry 37:512–518, 1998

Harris HE, Myers WC: Adolescents' misperceptions of the dangerousness of acetaminophen in overdose. Suicide Life Threat Behav 27:274–277, 1997

Hawton K: Why has suicide increased in young males? Crisis 19:119–124, 1998

Hawton K: Legislation on analgesic pack sizes: impact on suicidal behaviour. Suicide Life Threat Behav (in press)

Hawton K, Bancroft J, Catalan J, et al: Domiciliary and out-patient treatment of self-poisoning patients by medical and non-medical staff. Psychol Med 11:169–177, 1981

Hawton K, Cole D, O'Grady J, et al: Motivational aspects of deliberate self-poisoning in adolescents. Br J Psychiatry 141:286–291, 1982a

Hawton K, O'Grady J, Osborn M, et al: Adolescents who take overdoses: their characteristics, problems and contacts with helping agencies. Br J Psychiatry 140:118–123, 1982b

Hawton K, Fagg J, Platt S, et al: Factors associated with suicide after parasuicide in young people. BMJ 306:1641–1644, 1993

Hawton K, Arensman E, Townsend E, et al: Deliberate self-harm: systematic review of efficacy of psychosocial and pharmacological treatments in preventing repetition. BMJ 317:441–447, 1998

Hawton K, Kingsbury S, Steinhardt K, et al: Repetition of deliberate self-harm by adolescents: the role of psychological factors. J Adolesc 22:369–378, 1999

Hawton K, Fagg J, Simkin S, et al: Deliberate self-harm in adolescents in Oxford, 1985–1995. J Adolesc 23:47–55, 2000a

Hawton K, Townsend E, Arensman E, et al: Psychosocial versus pharmacological treatments for deliberate self harm (Cochrane Review), in The Cochrane Library 4. Oxford, England, Update Software, 2000b

Hawton K, Townsend E, Deeks J, et al: Effects of legislation restricting pack sizes of paracetamol and salicylate on self-poisoning in the United Kingdom: before and after study. BMJ 322:1203–1207, 2001

Haynes RH: Suicide and social response in Fiji: a historical survey. Br J Psychiatry 151:21–26, 1987

Hazell P, Lewin T: An evaluation of postvention following adolescent suicide. Suicide Life Threat Behav 23:101–109, 1993

Henley SHA: Bereavement following suicide: a review of the literature. Current Psychological Research and Reviews 3:53–61, 1984

Hirsch S: A critique of volunteer-staffed suicide prevention centers. Can J Psychiatry 26:406–410, 1981

Ho TP, Hung SF, Lee CC, et al: Characteristics of youth suicide in Hong Kong. Soc Psychiatry Psychiatr Epidemiol 30:107–112, 1995

Ho TP, Chao A, Yip P: Seasonal variation in suicides re-examined: no sex difference in Hong Kong and Taiwan. Acta Psychiatr Scand 95: 26–31, 1997

Holding TA: The BBC "Befrienders" series and its effects. Br J Psychiatry 124:470–472, 1974

Holding TA: Suicide and "The Befrienders." BMJ 3:751–752, 1975

Holinger PC, Offer D, Zola MA: A prediction model of suicide among youth. J Nerv Ment Dis 176:275–279, 1988

Isacsson G, Bergman U, Rich CL: Epidemiological data suggest antidepressants reduce suicide risk among depressives. J Affect Disord 41: 1–8, 1996

Isacsson G, Holmgren P, Druid H, et al: The utilization of antidepressants—a key issue in the prevention of suicide: an analysis of 5,281 suicides in Sweden during the period 1992–1994. Acta Psychiatr Scand 96:94–100, 1997

Jacobson B, Eklund G, Hamberger L, et al: Perinatal origin of adult self-destructive behavior. Acta Psychiatr Scand 76:364–371, 1987

Jeyaratnam J: Acute pesticide poisoning: a major global health problem. World Health Stat Q 43:139–144, 1990

Jobes DA, Berman AL, O'Carroll PW, et al: The Kurt Cobain suicide crisis: perspectives from research, public health, and the news media. Suicide Life Threat Behav 26:260–269, 1996

Johnson BA, Brent DA, Bridge J, et al: The familial aggregation of adolescent suicide attempts. Acta Psychiatr Scand 97:18–24, 1998

Johnson J, Weissman MM, Klerman GL: Panic disorder, comorbidity, and suicide attempts. Arch Gen Psychiatry 47:805–808, 1990

Kaltiala-Heino R, Rimpela M, Marttunen M, et al: Bullying, depression, and suicidal ideation in Finnish adolescents: school survey. BMJ 319:348–351, 1999

Kandel DB, Raveis VH, Davies M: Suicidal ideation in adolescence: depression, substance abuse, and other risk factors. Journal of Youth and Adolescence 20:289–309, 1991

Kevan SM: Perspectives on season of suicide: a review. Soc Sci Med 14:369–378, 1980

Kienhorst CW, Wolters WH, Diekstra RF, et al: A study of the frequency of suicidal behavior in children aged 5 to 14. J Child Psychol Psychiatry 28:153–165, 1987

Kienhorst CW, De Wilde EJ, Diekstra RF, et al: Differences between adolescent suicide attempters and depressed adolescents. Acta Psychiatr Scand 85:222–228, 1992

Kienhorst IC, De Wilde EJ, Diekstra RF, et al: Adolescents' image of their suicide attempt. J Am Acad Child Adolesc Psychiatry 34:623–628, 1995

King CA, Franzese R, Gargan S, et al: Suicide contagion among adolescents during acute psychiatric hospitalization. Psychiatr Serv 46:915–918, 1995

King RA, Riddle MA, Chappell PB, et al: Emergence of self-destructive phenomena in children and adolescents during fluoxetine treatment. J Am Acad Child Adolesc Psychiatry 30:179–186, 1991

King RA, Schwab-Stone M, Flisher AJ, et al: Psychosocial and risk behavior correlates of youth suicide attempts and suicidal ideation. J Am Acad Child Adolesc Psychiatry 40:837–846, 2001

Kingsbury S, Hawton K, Steinhardt K, et al: Do adolescents who take overdoses have specific psychological characteristics? A comparative study with psychiatric and community controls. J Am Acad Child Adolesc Psychiatry 38:1125–1131, 1999

Knowles D: On the tendency of volunteer helpers to give advice. Journal of Counseling Psychology 26:352–354, 1979

Kovacs M: The Children's Depression Inventory (CDI). Psychopharmacol Bull 21:995–998, 1985

Kreitman N: Parasuicide. Br J Psychiatry 115:746–747, 1969

Kruesi MJ, Grossman J, Pennington JM, et al: Suicide and violence prevention: parent education in the emergency department. J Am Acad Child Adolesc Psychiatry 38:250–255, 1999

Lerner MS, Clum GA: Treatment of suicide ideators: a problem-solving approach. Behavior Therapy 21:403–411, 1990

Lester D: Temporal variation in suicide and homicide. Am J Epidemiol 109:517–520, 1979

Letizia C, Kapik B, Flanders WD: Suicidal risk during controlled clinical investigations of fluvoxamine. J Clin Psychiatry 57:415–421, 1996

Lewinsohn PM, Rohde P, Seeley JR: Psychosocial risk factors for future adolescent suicide attempts. J Consult Clin Psychol 62:297–305, 1994

Lewinsohn PM, Rohde P, Seeley JR: Adolescent suicidal ideation and attempts: prevalence, risk factors, and clinical implications. Clinical Psychology: Science and Practice 3:25–46, 1996

Linehan MM, Armstrong HE, Suarez A, et al: Cognitive-behavioral treatment of chronically parasuicidal borderline patients. Arch Gen Psychiatry 48:1060–1064, 1991

Linehan MM, Heard HL, Armstrong HE: Naturalistic follow-up of a behavioral treatment for chronically parasuicidal borderline patients [published erratum appears in Arch Gen Psychiatry 51:422, 1994]. Arch Gen Psychiatry 50:971–974, 1993

Linehan MM, Tutek DA, Heard HL, et al: Interpersonal outcome of cognitive-behavioral treatment for chronically suicidal borderline patients. Am J Psychiatry 151:1771–1776, 1994

Litt IF, Cuskey WR, Rudd S: Emergency-room evaluation of the adolescent who attempts suicide: compliance with follow-up. Journal of Adolescent Health Care 4:106–108, 1983

Lock J, Steiner H: Gay, lesbian, and bisexual youth risks for emotional, physical, and social problems: results from a community-based survey. J Am Acad Child Adolesc Psychiatry 38:297–304, 1999

Lynskey M, Degenhardt L, Hall W: Cohort trends in youth suicide in Australia 1964–1997. Aust N Z J Psychiatry 34:408–412, 2000

Mann JJ, Kapur S: The emergence of suicidal ideation and behavior during antidepressant pharmacotherapy. Arch Gen Psychiatry 48:1027–1033, 1991

Mann JJ, Waternaux C, Haas GL, et al: Toward a clinical model of suicidal behavior in psychiatric patients. Am J Psychiatry 156:181–189, 1999

Marshall SE, Bird TG, Hart K, et al: Unified approach to the analysis of genetic variation in serotonergic pathways. Am J Med Genet 88:621–627, 1999

Marttunen MJ, Aro HM, Henriksson MM, et al: Mental disorders in adolescent suicide: DSM-III-R Axes I and II diagnoses in suicides among 13- to 19-year-olds in Finland. Arch Gen Psychiatry 48:834–839, 1991

Marttunen MJ, Aro HM, Lonnqvist JK: Precipitant stressors in adolescent suicide. J Am Acad Child Adolesc Psychiatry 32:1178–1183, 1993

Marttunen MJ, Henriksson MM, Aro HM, et al: Suicide among female adolescents: characteristics and comparison with males in the age group 13 to 22 years. J Am Acad Child Adolesc Psychiatry 34:1297–1307, 1995

May PA: Suicide and self-destruction among American Indian youths. Am Indian Alsk Native Ment Health Res 1:52–69, 1987

McClure GM: Changes in suicide in England and Wales, 1960–1997. Br J Psychiatry 176:64–67, 2000

Meares R, Mendelsohn FA, Milgrom-Friedman J: A sex difference in the seasonal variation of suicide rate: a single cycle for men, two cycles for women. Br J Psychiatry 138:321–325, 1981

Mercy JA, Kresnow MM, O'Carroll PW, et al: Is suicide contagious? A study of the relation between exposure to the suicidal behavior of others and nearly lethal suicide attempts. Am J Epidemiol 154:120–127, 2001

Michel K, Ballinari P, Bille-Brahe U, et al: Methods used for parasuicide: results of the WHO/EURO Multicenter Study on Parasuicide. Soc Psychiatry Psychiatr Epidemiol 35:156–163, 2000

Miller AL, Rathus JH, Linehan MM, et al: Dialectical behavior therapy adapted for suicidal adolescents. Journal of Practical Psychology and Behavioral Health 3:78–86, 1997

Miller KE, King CA, Shain BN, et al: Suicidal adolescents' perceptions of their family environment. Suicide Life Threat Behav 22:226–239, 1992

Miller S, Rotheram-Borus MJ, Piacentini J, et al: Successful Negotiation/Acting Positively (SNAP): A Brief Cognitive-Behavioral Therapy Manual for Adolescent Suicide Attempters and Their Families. New York, New York Psychiatric Institute, 1992

Mishara BL, Daigle MS: Help Lines and Crisis Intervention Services: Challenges for the Future in Suicide Prevention: Resources for the Millennium. Philadelphia, PA, Brunner/Mazel, 2000

Moens GF, Loysch MJ, van de Voorde H: The geographical pattern of methods of suicide in Belgium: implications for prevention. Acta Psychiatr Scand 77:320–327, 1988

Mohler B, Earls F: Trends in adolescent suicide: misclassification bias? Am J Public Health 91:150–153, 2001

Monk M, Warshauer ME: A methodologic problem in mortality studies of migrant populations. Journal of Chronic Diseases 31:347–352, 1978

Montgomery SA, Montgomery DB, Rani SJ, et al: Maintenance therapy in repeat suicidal behavior: a placebo controlled trial. Proceedings of the 10th International Congress of Suicide Prevention and Crisis Intervention, Ottawa, ON, 1979, pp 227–229

Montgomery SA, Dunner DL, Dunbar GC: Reduction of suicidal thoughts with paroxetine in comparison with reference antidepressants and placebo. Eur Neuropsychopharmacol 5:5–13, 1995

Morano CD, Cisler RA, Lemerond J: Risk factors for adolescent suicidal behavior: loss, insufficient familial support, and hopelessness. Adolescence 28:851–865, 1993

Motto JA: Suicide in male adolescents, in Suicide in the Young. Edited by Segdak HS, Ford AB, Rushforth NB. Boston, MA, John Wright PSG, 1984, pp 227–244

Murphy GE, Robins ER: Social factors in suicide. JAMA 199:303–308, 1967

Murphy GE, Wetzel RD: The lifetime risk of suicide in alcoholism. Arch Gen Psychiatry 47:383–392, 1990

Myers WC: What treatments do we have for children and adolescents who have killed? Bull Am Acad Psychiatry Law 20:47–58, 1992

National Center for Health Statistics: National Center for Injury Prevention and Control, Office of Statistics and Programming. Web-based Injury Statistics Query and Reporting System (WISQARS). Available at: http://www.cdc.gov/ncipc/wisqars. Accessed August 1, 1999

National Center for Health Statistics, Centers for Disease Control and Prevention: Death Rates for 72 Selected Causes, by 5-Year Age Groups, Race, and Sex: United States, 1979–1998. Worktable GMWK 291, 2000. Available at: www.cdc.gov/nchs/datawh/statab/unpubd/mortabs.htm

National Center for Health Statistics, Centers for Disease Control and Prevention: Deaths: final data for 1999. Natl Vital Stat Rep 49(8), 2001a

National Center for Health Statistics, Centers for Disease Control and Prevention: Deaths: preliminary data for 2000. National Vital Statistics Report 49(12), 2001b

National Crime Records Bureau: Accidental deaths and suicides in India 1999. Delhi, Ministry of Home Affairs, Government of India, supplied upon written request to http://ncrb.nic.in/ncrb.htm. Contacted September 1, 2001

Neeleman J, Wessely S: Ethnic minority suicide: a small area geographical study in south London. Psychol Med 29:429–436, 1999

Neeleman J, Wessely S, Lewis G: Suicide acceptability in African- and white Americans: the role of religion. J Nerv Ment Dis 186:12–16, 1998

New Zealand Health Information Service: Health statistics: youth suicide rates for 1988–1999. Available at http://www.nzhis.govt.nz/stats/youthsuicide.html. Updated July 25, 2001. Accessed September 3, 2001

Nielsen DA, Goldman D, Virkkunen M, et al: Suicidality and 5-hydroxyindoleacetic acid concentration associated with a tryptophan hydroxylase polymorphism. Arch Gen Psychiatry 51:34–38, 1994

Nielsen DA, Virkkunen M, Lappalainen J, et al: A tryptophan hydroxylase gene marker for suicidality and alcoholism. Arch Gen Psychiatry 55:593–602, 1998

Nordstrom P, Samuelsson M, Åsberg M, et al: CSF 5-HIAA predicts suicide risk after attempted suicide. Suicide Life Threat Behav 24:1–9, 1994

Offer D, Howard KI, Schonert KA, et al: To whom do adolescents turn for help? Differences between disturbed and nondisturbed adolescents. J Am Acad Child Adolesc Psychiatry 30:623–630, 1991

Ohara K, Nagai M, Tani K, et al: Functional polymorphism of -141C Ins/Del in the dopamine D2 receptor gene promoter and schizophrenia. Psychiatry Res 81:117–123, 1998

Ohberg A, Vuori E, Klaukka T, et al: Antidepressants and suicide mortality. J Affect Disord 50:225–233, 1998

Oldham JM, Riba MB: Introduction to the Review of Psychiatry Series, in PTSD in Children and Adolescents, Vol 20. Edited by Eth S. Washington, DC, American Psychiatric Press, 1998, pp xii–xvi

Olfson M, Marcus SC, Pincus HA, et al: Antidepressant prescribing practices of outpatient psychiatrists. Arch Gen Psychiatry 55:310–316, 1998

Oquendo MA, Mann JJ: The biology of impulsivity and suicidality. Psychiatr Clin North Am 23:11–25, 2000

Otto U: Suicidal acts by children and adolescents: a follow-up study. Acta Psychiatr Scand Suppl 233:7–123, 1972

Parker G, Gao F, Machin D: Seasonality of suicide in Singapore: data from the equator. Psychol Med 31:549–553, 2001

Pfeffer CR, Klerman GL, Hurt SW, et al: Suicidal children grow up: demographic and clinical risk factors for adolescent suicide attempts. J Am Acad Child Adolesc Psychiatry 30:609–616, 1991

Pfeffer CR, Jiang H, Kakuma T: Child-Adolescent Suicidal Potential Index (CASPI): a screen for risk for early onset suicidal behavior. Psychological Assessment 12:304–318, 2000

Phillips DP: The influence of suggestion on suicide: substantive and theoretical implications of the Werther effect. American Sociological Review 39:340–354, 1974

Phillips DP: Suicide, motor vehicle fatalities, and the mass media: evidence toward a theory of suggestion. American Journal of Sociology 84:1150–1174, 1979

Phillips DP: Airplane accidents, murder and the mass media: towards a theory of imitation and suggestion. Social Forces 58:1001–1004, 1980

Phillips DP: Teenage and adult temporal fluctuations in suicide and auto fatalities, in Suicide in the Young. Edited by Sudak HS, Ford AB, Rushforth NB. Littleton, MA, John Wright PSG, 1984, pp 69–80

Piacentini J, Rotheram-Borus MJ, Trautman P, et al: Psychosocial correlates of treatment compliance in adolescent suicide attempters. Presented at the meeting of the Association for Advancement of Behavior Therapy, New York, May 1991

Platt S, Bille-Brahe U, Kerkhof A, et al: Parasuicide in Europe: the WHO/EURO Multicenter Study on Parasuicide, I: introduction and preliminary analysis for 1989. Acta Psychiatr Scand 85:97–104, 1992

Reid WH: Promises, promises: don't rely on patients' no-suicide/no-violence "contracts." Journal of Practical Psychiatry and Behavioral Health 4:316–318, 1998

Reifman A, Windle M: Adolescent suicidal behaviors as a function of depression, hopelessness, alcohol use, and social support: a longitudinal investigation. Am J Community Psychol 23:329–354, 1995

Reinherz HZ, Giaconia RM, Silverman AB, et al: Early psychosocial risks for adolescent suicidal ideation and attempts. J Am Acad Child Adolesc Psychiatry 34:599–611, 1995

Remafedi G, French S, Story M, et al: The relationship between suicide risk and sexual orientation: results of a population-based study. Am J Public Health 88:57–60, 1998

Renaud J, Brent DA, Birmaher B, et al: Suicide in adolescents with disruptive disorders. J Am Acad Child Adolesc Psychiatry 38:846–851, 1999

Renouf AG, Kovacs M: Concordance between mothers' reports and children's self-reports of depressive symptoms: a longitudinal study. J Am Acad Child Adolesc Psychiatry 33:208–216, 1994

Reynolds WM: Suicidal Ideation Questionnaire (SIQ). Odessa, FL, Psychological Assessment Resources, 1987

Reynolds WM: A school-based procedure for the identification of adolescents at risk for suicidal behaviors. Family Community Health 14:64–75, 1991

Rigby K, Slee P: Suicidal ideation among adolescent school children, involvement in bully victim problems, and perceived social support. Suicide Life Threat Behav 29:119–130, 1999

Rihmer Z, Rutz W, Pihlgren H: Depression and suicide on Gotland: an intensive study of all suicides before and after a depression-training program for general practitioners. J Affect Disord 35:147–152, 1995

Rihmer Z, Rutz W, Pihlgren H, et al: Decreasing tendency of seasonality in suicide may indicate lowering rate of depressive suicides in the population. Psychiatry Res 81:233–240, 1998

Robins E, Murphy GE, Wilkinson RH, et al: Some clinical considerations in the prevention of suicide based on a study of 134 successful suicides. Am J Public Health 49:888–899, 1959

Rogers J, Sheldon A, Barwick C, et al: Help for families of suicide: survivors support program. Can J Psychiatry 27:444–449, 1982

Rohn RD, Sarles RM, Kenny TJ, et al: Adolescents who attempt suicide. J Pediatr 90:636–638, 1977

Rotheram-Borus MJ, Trautman PD, Dopkins SC, et al: Cognitive style and pleasant activities among female adolescent suicide attempters. J Consult Clin Psychol 58:554–561, 1990

Rotheram-Borus MJ, Piacentini J, Cantwell C, et al: The 18-month impact of an emergency-room intervention for adolescent female suicide attempters. J Consult Clin Psychol 68:1081–1093, 2000

Rothschild AJ, Locke CA: Reexposure to fluoxetine after serious suicide attempts by three patients: the role of akathisia. J Clin Psychiatry 52: 491–493, 1991

Roy A, Nielsen DA, Rylander G, et al: The genetics of suicidal behavior, in The International Handbook of Suicide and Attempted Suicide. Edited by Hawton K, van Heeringen K. Chichester, England, Wiley, 2000, pp 209–221

Rujescu D, Giegling I, Sato T, et al: A polymorphism in the promoter of the serotonin transporter gene is not associated with suicidal behavior. Psychiatr Genet 11:169–172, 2001

Rushton JL, Whitmire JT: Pediatric stimulant and selective serotonin reuptake inhibitor prescription trends: 1992 to 1998. Arch Pediatr Adolesc Med 155:560–565, 2001

Rutz W, von Knorring L, Walinder J: Long-term effects of an educational program for general practitioners given by the Swedish Committee for the Prevention and Treatment of Depression. Acta Psychiatr Scand 85:83–88, 1992

Rutz W, von Knorring AL, Pihlgren H, et al: An educational project on depression and its consequences: is the frequency of major depression among Swedish men underrated, resulting in high suicidality? Primary Care Psychiatry 1:59–63, 1995

Ryan ND, Varma D: Child and adolescent mood disorders—experience with serotonin-based therapies. Biol Psychiatry 44:336–340, 1998

Safer DJ: Changing patterns of psychotropic medications prescribed by child psychiatrists in the 1990s. J Child Adolesc Psychopharmacol 7:267–274, 1997

Salk L, Lipsitt LP, Sturner WQ, et al: Relationship of maternal and perinatal conditions to eventual adolescent suicide. Lancet 1:624–627, 1985

Schmidtke A, Hafner H: Facilitation of suicide motivation and suicidal behavior by fictional models: sequelae of the television series "Death of a Student." Nervenarzt 57:502–510, 1986

Schmidtke A, Bille-Brahe U, DeLeo D, et al: Attempted suicide in Europe: rates, trends and sociodemographic characteristics of suicide attempters during the period 1989–1992: results of the WHO/EURO Multicenter Study on Parasuicide. Acta Psychiatr Scand 93:327–338, 1996

Schulsinger R, Kety S, Rosenthal D, et al: A family study of suicide, in Origins, Prevention and Treatment of Affective Disorders. Edited by Schou M, Stromgren E. New York, Academic Press, 1979, pp 277–287

Sellar C, Hawton K, Goldacre MJ: Self-poisoning in adolescents: hospital admissions and deaths in the Oxford region 1980–85. Br J Psychiatry 156:866–870, 1990

Shaffer D: Suicide in childhood and early adolescence. J Child Psychol Psychiatry 15:275–291, 1974

Shaffer D, Craft L: Methods of adolescent suicide prevention. J Clin Psychiatry 60 (suppl 2):70–74, 1999

Shaffer D, Garland A, Gould M, et al: Preventing teenage suicide: a critical review. J Am Acad Child Adolesc Psychiatry 27:675–687, 1988

Shaffer D, Vieland V, Garland A, et al: Adolescent suicide attempters: response to suicide-prevention programs. JAMA 264:3151–3155, 1990

Shaffer D, Garland A, Vieland V, et al: The impact of curriculum-based suicide prevention programs for teenagers. J Am Acad Child Adolesc Psychiatry 30:588–596, 1991

Shaffer D, Gould MS, Fisher P, et al: Psychiatric diagnosis in child and adolescent suicide. Arch Gen Psychiatry 53:339–348, 1996

Shaffer D, Fisher P, Lucas CP, et al: NIMH Diagnostic Interview Schedule for Children Version IV (NIMH DISC-IV): description, differences from previous versions, and reliability of some common diagnoses. J Am Acad Child Adolesc Psychiatry 39:28–38, 2000

Shneidman E, Farberow N: Clues to Suicide. New York, McGraw-Hill, 1957

Silverstone T, Romans S, Hunt N, et al: Is there a seasonal pattern of relapse in bipolar affective disorders? A dual northern and southern hemisphere cohort study. Br J Psychiatry 167:58–60, 1995

Simmons JT, Comstock BS, Franklin JL: Prevention/intervention programs for suicidal adolescents. Prepared for the Prevention and Intervention Work Group of the Secretary of Health and Human Services' Task Force on Youth Suicide, Oakland, CA, June 1986

Simon TR, Crosby AE: Suicide planning among high-school students who report attempting suicide. Suicide Life Threat Behav 30:213–221, 2000

Slaiku KA, Tulkin SR, Speer DC: Process and outcome in the evaluation of telephone counseling referrals. J Consult Clin Psychol 43:700–707, 1975

Smith K, Crawford S: Suicidal behavior among "normal" high-school students. Suicide Life Threat Behav 16:313–325, 1986

Sonneck G, Etzersdorfer E, Nagel-Kuess S: Imitative suicide on the Viennese subway. Soc Sci Med 38:453–457, 1994

Sourander A, Helstela L, Haavisto A, et al: Suicidal thoughts and attempts among adolescents: a longitudinal 8-year follow-up study. J Affect Disord 63:59–66, 2001

Spirito A, Overholser J, Ashworth S, et al: Evaluation of a suicide-awareness curriculum for high-school students. J Am Acad Child Adolesc Psychiatry 27:705–711, 1988

Spirito A, Brown L, Overholser J, et al: Attempted suicide in adolescence: a review and critique of the literature. Clin Psychol Rev 9:335–363, 1989

Spirito A, Overholser J, Hart K: Cognitive characteristics of adolescent suicide attempters. J Am Acad Child Adolesc Psychiatry 30:604–608, 1991

Stanley EJ, Barter JT: Adolescent suicidal behavior. Am J Orthopsychiatry 40:87–93, 1970

Statham DJ, Heath AC, Madden PA, et al: Suicidal behavior: an epidemiological and genetic study. Psychol Med 28:839–855, 1998

Statistics Canada, Health Statistics Division: Suicides Canada 1950–1998. Ottawa, Ontario, Statistics Canada, 2001, Sections 1, 2, and 3, p 2

Statistics Finland: StatFin Tilastopalvelu Valintaohjelma. Youth suicide information for 1988–1999, supplied upon written request to Kirjasto.tilastokeskus@stat.fi. Contacted September 10, 2001

Statistics Sweden, Division of Centre of Epidemiology, National Board of Health and Welfare: Cause of death registry, supplied upon written request to Statistics Sweden at http://www.sos.se/epc/dorseng.htm. Contacted September 1, 2001

Steer RA, Rissmiller DJ, Ranieri WF, et al: Dimensions of suicidal ideation in psychiatric inpatients. Behav Res Ther 31:229–236, 1993

Stein D, Apter A, Ratzoni G, et al: Association between multiple suicide attempts and negative affects in adolescents. J Am Acad Child Adolesc Psychiatry 37:488–494, 1998

Stuart R: Helping Couples Change: A Social Learning Approach to Marital Therapy. New York, Guilford, 1980

Sudak HS, Sawyer JB, Spring GK, et al: High referral success rates in a crisis center. Hospital and Community Psychiatry 28:530–532, 1977

Swanston HY, Nunn KP, Oates RK, et al: Hoping and coping in young people who have been sexually abused. Eur Child Adolesc Psychiatry 8:134–142, 1999

Swedo SE: Postdischarge therapy of hospitalized adolescent suicide attempters. J Adolesc 10:541–544, 1989

Szabo CP, Blanche MJ: Seasonal variation in mood disorder presentation: further evidence of this phenomenon in a South African sample. J Affect Disord 33:209–214, 1995

Tatman SM, Greene AL, Karr LC: Use of the Suicide Probability Scale (SPS) with adolescents. Suicide Life Threat Behav 23:188–203, 1993

Taylor EA, Stansfeld SA: Children who poison themselves, I: a clinical comparison with psychiatric controls. Br J Psychiatry 145:127–132, 1984

Teicher MH, Glod C, Cole JO: Emergence of intense suicidal preoccupation during fluoxetine treatment. Am J Psychiatry 147:207–210, 1990

Tondo L, Jamison KR, Baldessarini RJ: Effect of lithium maintenance on suicidal behavior in major mood disorders. Ann N Y Acad Sci 836:339–351, 1997

Trautman P, Rotheram-Borus MJ: Cognitive therapy with children and adolescents, in American Psychiatric Press Review of Psychiatry, Vol 7. Edited by Frances AJ, Hales RE. Washington, DC, American Psychiatric Press, 1988, pp 307–323

Trautman PD, Shaffer D: Treatment of child and adolescent suicide attempters, in Suicide in the Young. Edited by Sudak HS, Ford AB, Rushforth NB. Boston, MA, John Wright PSG, 1984, pp 307–323

Trautman PD, Shaffer D: Pediatric management of suicidal behavior. Pediatr Ann 18:134–143, 1989

United Kingdom Office for National Statistics: Mortality statistics, injury and poisoning: review of the Registrar General on Deaths Attributed to England and Wales. Available at www.statistics.gov.uk. Accessed September 1, 2000

Vajda J, Steinbeck K: Factors associated with repeat suicide attempts among adolescents. Aust N Z J Psychiatry 34:437–445, 2000

van der Sande SR, van Rooijen L, Buskens E, et al: Intensive inpatient and community intervention versus routine care after attempted suicide: a randomized controlled intervention study. Br J Psychiatry 171:35–41, 1997

Velez CN, Cohen P: Suicidal behavior and ideation in a community sample of children: maternal and youth reports. J Am Acad Child Adolesc Psychiatry 27:349–356, 1988

Velting DM, Gould MS: Suicide contagion, in Annual Review of Suicidology. Edited by Maris R, Canetto S, Silverman MM. New York, Guilford, 1997, pp 96–136

Verkes RJ, Van der Mast RC, Hengeveld MW, et al: Reduction by paroxetine of suicidal behavior in patients with repeated suicide attempts but not major depression. Am J Psychiatry 155:543–547, 1998a

Verkes RJ, Van der Mast RC, Kerkhof AJ, et al: Platelet serotonin, monoamine oxidase activity, and [3H]paroxetine binding related to impulsive suicide attempts and borderline personality disorder. Biol Psychiatry 43:740–746, 1998b

Vieland V, Whittle B, Garland A, et al: The impact of curriculum-based suicide prevention programs for teenagers: an 18-month follow-up. J Am Acad Child Adolesc Psychiatry 30:811–815, 1991

Vijayakumar L, Rajkumar S: Are risk factors for suicide universal? A case-control study in India. Acta Psychiatr Scand 99:407–411, 1999

Warshaw MG, Dolan RT, Keller MB: Suicidal behavior in patients with current or past panic disorder: five years of prospective data from the Harvard/Brown Anxiety Research Program. Am J Psychiatry 157:1876–1878, 2000

Wasserman IM: Imitation and suicide: a reexamination of the Werther effect. American Sociological Review 49:427–436, 1984

Waterhouse J, Platt S: General hospital admission in the management of parasuicide: a randomized controlled trial. Br J Psychiatry 156:236–242, 1990

Weissman MM, Klerman GL, Markowitz JS, et al: Suicidal ideation and suicide attempts in panic disorder and attacks. N Engl J Med 321:1209–1214, 1989

White HC: Self-poisoning in adolescents. Br J Psychiatry 124:24–35, 1974

Wichstrom L: Predictors of adolescent suicide attempts: a nationally representative longitudinal study of Norwegian adolescents. J Am Acad Child Adolesc Psychiatry 39:603–610, 2000

World Health Organization: World Health Statistics Annual 1987–1995. Geneva, World Health Organization, 1987–1995

World Health Organization and WHOSIS (WHO Statistical Information System): Online version of the World Health Statistics Annual 1997–1999: Mortality Data. Geneva, World Health Organization, 2000. Available at www.who.int/whosis.

World Health Organization: Suicide rates and absolute numbers of suicide by country. Available at http://www.who.int/mental_health/Topic_Suicide/suicide1.html. Updated July 14, 2001. Accessed September 1, 2001

Yip PS, Chao A, Ho TP: A re-examination of seasonal variation in suicides in Australia and New Zealand. J Affect Disord 47:141–150, 1998

Yip PS, Chao A, Chiu CW: Seasonal variation in suicides: diminished or vanished: experience from England and Wales, 1982–1996. Br J Psychiatry 177:366–369, 2000

Index

*Page numbers printed in **boldface type** refer to tables or figures.*

Antidepressants *(continued)*
    need for research on, 96–97
    optimizing initial treatment, 93
    other drugs, 80
    selective serotonin reuptake
        inhibitors, 75–79
    switching between, 93–94
    for treatment-resistant
        depression, 93–95
    tricyclic (TCAs), 75, 79–80
        for bipolar depression, 82
        for comorbid depression
            and attention-deficit/
            hyperactivity disorder,
            80
        for maintenance therapy, 91
        response to, 79–80
        selective serotonin reuptake
            inhibitors and, 79, 80, 95
Antihypertensive agents, 79
Antipsychotics
    interaction with selective sero-
        tonin reuptake inhibitors,
        79
    for psychotic depression, 81
Anxiety disorders, 115
    behavioral inhibition and, 20
    bipolar disorder and, 108
    depression and, 9, 48, 84
    selective serotonin reuptake
        inhibitors for, 75
    suicidality and, 138, 141, 143
Appetite disturbances
    depression-related, 7
    selective serotonin reuptake
        inhibitor–induced, 77
Attention-deficit/hyperactivity
    disorder (ADHD), 106
    depression and, 80, 83, 85, 97
    family studies of, 112
    irritability and, 114, 115

mania and, 108, 109, 120
    suicidality and, 138
Attentional problems, 4, 108

Barbiturate overdose, 142
Beck Depression Inventory (BDI),
    13, **14**
Behavioral activation, 77, 112
Behavioral disturbances, 1, 9
Behavioral problem-solving
    therapy, 42
Behaviorally inhibited tempera-
    ment, 20
Benzodiazepines, 79
Biological correlates of depres-
    sion, 19–23
    brain anatomy, 22
    genetics, 19–20
    neuroendocrine factors, 21
    neurotransmitter studies,
        21–22
    sleep disturbances, 22–23
    temperament, 20
Bipolar disorder, 105–121
    age at onset of, 107, 109
    assessment of, 113–117
        interviews, 114–116
        rating scales, 116–117
    bipolar II disorder, 82, 107
    classical, 111
    comorbidity with, 108–109
    complicated, 111
    definitional problems related
        to, 105–106
    epidemiology of, 106–108
    family studies of, 112–113
    follow-up for, 119–120
    genetic subtypes of, 113
    neuroimaging in, 110
    not otherwise specified,
        113–114

obstetrical complications and, 109–110
outcomes of, 120
pharmacotherapy for bipolar depression, 82–83, 97
phenomenology and differential diagnosis of, 110–112
psychosis and, 110–111
rapid cycling, 105
suicide and, 134
treatment of, 118–119
Bisexual youth, 25
Borderline personality disorder
dialectical behavior therapy for suicidal adolescents with features of, 62
differentiation from mania, 111
Brain anatomy
in bipolar disorder, 110
in depression, 22
Bright-light therapy, 81
Bupropion, 75, 80, 85
for bipolar depression, 82, 83
for comorbid depression and attention-deficit/hyperactivity disorder, 83, 97

CAPA (Child and Adolescent Psychiatric Assessment), **11, 18**
Carbamazepine, 79, 82
Catecholamines, 22
CBCL (Child Behavior Checklist), 116
CBT. *See* Cognitive-behavioral therapy
CDI (Children's Depression Inventory), 13, **14,** 41
CDRS (Children's Depression Rating Scale), 13, **14,** 41, **74,** 76, 92

Center for Epidemiologic Studies Depression Scale (CES-D), **14,** 51
CGI-S (Clinical Global Impression Improvement subscale), 76, 92
Child abuse, 24, 141
Child and Adolescent Psychiatric Assessment (CAPA), **11, 18**
Child Behavior Checklist (CBCL), 116
Children's Attributional Style Questionnaire, 50
Children's Depression Inventory (CDI), 13, **14,** 41
Children's Depression Rating Scale (CDRS), 13, **14,** 41, **74,** 76, 92
Children's Interview for Psychiatric Syndromes (ChIPS), **12**
m-Chlorophenylpiperazine, 22
Citalopram, 78, 79, 85
Clinical course of mood episode, 27–28
Clinical Global Impression Improvement subscale (CGI-S), 76, 92
Clinical presentations of depression, 2–6
family conflict, 4
increasing illicit substance abuse, 5
mood symptoms, 3
school problems, 3–4
somatic symptoms, 5–6
suicidal crises, 5
Clomipramine, intravenous, 92, 95
Cluster suicides, 147, 157–158

Hormonal factors, 21
Hospitalization of suicidal
    patients, 57, 84, 150
    indications for, 150, **151**
    poor treatment compliance
        after, 59
Hot lines for suicide prevention,
    156–157
5-Hydroxyindoleacetic acid
    (5-HIAA), 144–147
L-5-Hydroxytryptophan, 22
Hyperactivity, 1, 108. *See also*
    Attention-deficit/hyper-
    activity disorder
Hypersomnia
    depression-related, 7
    SSRI–induced, 77
Hypomania, 28, 82, 105–106
    epidemiology of, 107–108
    induced by bright-light
        therapy, 82
    induced by selective serotonin
        reuptake inhibitors, 77
    seasonality of, 134
Hyponatremia, 77

Imipramine, 76, 79, 80
Impulsivity, 84, 141, 142, 158
Incidence rates
    for bipolar disorder, 106
    for depression, 17–19
Insomnia
    antidepressants for, 80
    depression-related, 22
    SSRI–induced, 77
Interpersonal psychotherapy
    (IPT), 38, 52–54, 86
    adaptation for depressed
        adolescents, 52–54
    compared with cognitive-
        behavioral therapy, 53–54

efficacy studies of, 52
    goals of, 52
Interview Schedule for Children
    and Adolescents (ISCA), **12**
Interviews, diagnostic
    for bipolar disorder, 114–116
    for depression, 7–8
IPT. *See* Interpersonal psycho-
    therapy
Irritability, 3, 4, 7, 108, 110,
    114–115
ISCA (Interview Schedule for
    Children and Adolescents),
    12
Isotretinoin, 6

Jitteriness, 77

K-SADS (Schedule for Affective
    Disorders and Schizophrenia
    for School-Aged Children),
    10, **11**, **14**, **18**, 44, 51

Learned helplessness, 23, 24
Learning disabilities, 9
Lesbian youth, 25, 138–139
Lithium
    for antidepressant augmenta-
        tion, 94
    for bipolar disorder, 82, 83,
        118–119
    continuation therapy with,
        87
    maintenance therapy with, 91
    for pure mania, 111
    for suicidality, 151
Loss events, 24

Magnetic resonance
    spectroscopy, in bipolar
    disorder, 110

Organic mood disorder, 111
Organophosphate ingestion, 142
Outcomes
    of depression, 16
        impact of comorbidity on,
            9–10
        long-term sequelae, 28
        predictors in adolescents, 45
    of mania, 120

Panic disorder, 112
Paraquat ingestion, 142
Parasuicide, 139–140
Parents
    child's conflicts with, 4
    impact of maladaptive
        parenting behavior, 26
    interviews with, 8
    involvement in Coping With
        Depression Course, 44–45
    parent-child disagreement
        during diagnostic
        assessment, 8–9
    psychopathology in, 9, 26, 86
Paroxetine, 76–78, 85
Peer environments, 26
PENN Prevention Program,
    49–51
Personality disorders, 28, 84, 86
Pervasive developmental
    disorder, 109, 115
Pessimism, 23
Pharmacotherapy for depression,
    73–97
    acute phase treatment, 74–86
        for atypical depression, 81
        for bipolar depression,
            82–83, 97
        for comorbid conditions
            and suicidality, 83–84
        other antidepressants, 80

for psychotic depression,
    80–81
for seasonal affective
    disorder, 81–82
selective serotonin reuptake
    inhibitors, 75–79
summary and recommen-
    dations for, 84–86
tricyclic antidepressants,
    79–80
continuation therapy, 74, 86–88
definitions of response to, **74**
goals of, 73–74
maintenance therapy, 74, 88–91
noncompliance with, 92
nonresponse to, 92
for treatment-resistant
    depression, 93–95
    augmenting or combining
        treatments, 94–95
    optimizing initial
        treatments, 93
    switching strategies, 93–94
Pharmacotherapy for suicidality,
    151
Phenobarbital, 6
Physical abuse, 24, 141
Physician education programs
    for suicide prevention,
    155
Polycystic ovary disease, 119
Polypharmacy, 85
Posttraumatic stress disorder
    (PTSD), 55, 84
Poverty, 17, 25
Pregnancy complications
    bipolar disorder and, 109–110
    suicidality and, 144
Prevalence rates
    for depression, 17, **18,** 73
    for suicidality, 57

Restlessness, 77
Reynolds Adolescent Depression
    Scale (RADS), **14**
Risk factors for depression, 17,
    19–26
    biological correlates, 19–23
    psychological correlates, 23–25
    social/environmental
        correlates, 25–26
Risperidone, 81

Schedule for Affective Disorders
    and Schizophrenia, Lifetime
    Version (SADS-L), 108
Schedule for Affective Disorders
    and Schizophrenia for
    School-Aged Children
    (K-SADS), 10, **11, 14, 18,** 44,
    51
Schizophrenia, 143
School-based services
    for early recognition of
        depression, 3
    for evaluation of somatic
        symptoms, 6
    for primary prevention of
        depression in adolescents,
        51
    for suicide prevention, 157
School problems, 3–4, 85
Seasonal affective disorder, 81–82
Selective serotonin reuptake
    inhibitors (SSRIs), 75–79,
    84–85
    for anxiety disorders, 75
    augmentation of, 80
    for bipolar depression, 82, 83
    discontinuation of, 77–78
    dosage and administration of,
        76, 77, 85
    drug interactions, 78–79, 95

for maintenance therapy, 91
    mechanism of action of, 75
    nonresponse to, 77, 78, 96
    for obsessive-compulsive
        disorder, 75
    overdose of, 75
    pharmacogenetic studies of, 78
    pharmacokinetic studies of, 78
    protein binding of, 79
    response to, 75–76, 96
    side effects of, 77
    suicidality and, 57, 137,
        148–149
    switching to another drug
        from, 94–96
Self-control therapy, 42–43
Self-esteem problems, 86
Self-injurious behavior, 5, 60.
    See also Suicidality
Self-reports
    of depressive symptomatol-
        ogy, 8–9
    of suicidality, 153–154
Serotonergic dysfunction
    aggressivity and, 145
    depression and, 22
    suicidality and, 144–147
Serotonin syndrome, 79
Sertraline, 78, 79, 85
Sex differences
    in depression risk, 17, 19, 21
    in suicidality, 129–131, 133,
        133, 135
Sex hormones, 21
Sexual abuse, 24, 84, 141
Sexual behavior, 4
Sexual dysfunction, 77
Sexual identity, 25, 138–139
Sibling conflicts, 4
Sleep disturbances
    depression-related, 22–23